Recent Results in Cancer Research

155

Springer
Berlin
Heidelberg
New York
Barcelona
Hong Kong
London
Milan
Paris
Singapore
Tokyo

J. Lange J. R. Siewert (Eds.)

Esophageal Carcinoma

State of the Art

With 59 Figures and 37 Tables

Springer

Prof. Dr. med. Jochen Lange
Kantonsspital St. Gallen
Klinik für Chirurgie
CH-9007 St. Gallen

Prof. Dr. med. J.R. Siewert
Chirurgische Klinik und Poliklinik
Klinikum rechts der Isar
Ismaninger Straße 22
81675 München, Germany

ISBN-13:978-3-642-64044-5
ISSN 0080-0015

Library of Congress Cataloging-in-Publication Data.
Die Deutsche Bibliothek - CIP-Einheitsaufnahme
Esophageal carcinoma: state of the art / J. Lange; J.R. Siewert (ed.). -
Berlin; Heidelberg; New York; Barcelona; Hong Kong; London; Milan; Paris; Singapore; Tokyo: Springer, 2000
(Recent results in cancer research; 155)
ISBN-13:978-3-642-64044-5 e-ISBN-13:978-3-642-59600-1
DOI: 10.1007/978-3-642-59600-1

Softcover reprint of the hardcover 1st edition 2000

Production: PRO EDIT GmbH, 69126 Heidelberg, Germany
Typesetting: K+V Fotosatz GmbH, 64743 Beerfelden, Germany

SPIN 10702531 21/3133-5 4 3 2 1 0 - Printed on acid-free paper

Preface

The Symposium "Esophageal Carcinoma – State of the Art" has aroused very great interest. The numerous enquiries have caused us to publish the congress proceedings in the present volume. Particular attention was paid to current topical problems. One of the areas on which the present volume focuses is the epidemiology and pathology of esophageal adenocarcinoma. Compared to squamous epithelial carcinoma, this is increasing in incidence in Europe. Modern diagnostic methods are described such as laser-induced fluorescence spectroscopy or the optical coherence endoscopic technique. The latter enables normal mucosa to be distinguished from dysplastic or malignant lesions, in contrast to conventional endoscopy. As in other tumors of the gastrointestinal tract, neoadjuvant therapy is becoming of increasing importance. Since the indication crucially depends on the tumor stage, two contributions deal with postoperative staging, with the diagnostic reliability of the individual techniques and new methods such as endoluminal MRI. There is no doubt that neoadjuvant chemotherapy is indicated in tumors which are irresectable and in tumor stages in which resectability is uncertain. However, to what extent it should also be applied in the resectable stage will be discussed in the individual contributions both for adenocarcinoma and for squamous epithelial carcinoma. In the meantime, surgical treatment of esophageal carcinoma has been largely standardized. Differences with regard to radicality are still found in the extent of lymphadenectomy, especially in inclusion of cervical lymph nodes.

Since cervical esophageal carcinoma is a special entity with regard to pretreatment and surgical technique, it gets a chapter of its own.

The greatest problem in replacing the esophagus with stomach tube prosthesis or colon interponate is still the problem of dehiscence in the region of the cervical anastomosis.

The various methods will therefore be dealt with in extra chapters. New methods such as gastric conditioning or fundus rotation plasty will also be described.

New minimally invasive methods for treatment of early tumor stages which correspond to the current trend are photodynamic treatment and endoscopic mucosectomy. The technique, indication and the therapeutic effectiveness are described in the relevant sections.

Even though it is not possible to treat the topic of esophageal carcinoma exhaustively in congress proceedings, it has nevertheless been possible to provide an overview of current topics in esophageal surgery.

Autumn, 1999 The Editors

Contents

List of Contributors*

Alderson, D.[193]
Bartels, H.[89]
Blazeby, J. M.[193]
Bohorfoush, A. G.[55]
Bonavina, L.[119]
Büchler, M. W.[145]
Chen, K.[151]
Cheng, B.[151]
Cseke, L.[161]
Ell, C.[175]
Fantin, A. C.[63]
Farndon, J. R.[193]
Feith, M.[42]
Forastiere, A. A.[97]
Gabbert, H. E.[15]
Gao, S.[151]
Gossner, L.[175]
Heitmiller, R. F.[97]
Horváth, Ö. P.[161]
Imai, Y.[73]
Kato, H.[123]
Kelsen, D. P.[105]
Kitajima, M.[73]
Kleinberg, L.[97]
Kriwanek, S.[113]
Lambert, R.[183]
Lukács, L.[161]
Meyenberger, C.[63]
Mueller, J.[29]
Ozawa, S.[73]
Pera, M.[1]
Peracchia, A.[119]
Roka, R.[113]
Roka, S.[113]
Ruol, A.[119]
Sarbia, M.[15]
Schilling, M. K.[145]
Siewert, J. R.[29, 42, 89]
Stein, H. J.[42, 89, 119]
Suwa, T.[73]
Tachimori, Y.[123]
Tu, Z.[151]
Urschel, J. D.[135]
Watanabe, H.[123]
Werner, M.[29]
Zahurak, M.[97]

* The address of the principal author is given on the first page of each contribution.
[1] Page on which contribution begins.

Epidemiology of Esophageal Cancer, Especially Adenocarcinoma of the Esophagus and Esophagogastric Junction

M. Pera

Department of Surgery, Service of Digestive and General Surgery,
Hospital Clinic y Provincial, University of Barcelona Medical School,
Villarroel 170, 08036 Barcelona, Spain

Abstract

The incidence of adenocarcinoma of the esophagus and esophagogastric junction (EGJ) has been increasing over the past 15 years in western countries. Surgical series and population-based studies show that, by 1994, adenocarcinomas of the esophagus accounted for half of all esophageal cancer among white men. The causes of this increase in incidence remain to be elucidated. Esophageal adenocarcinomas and a portion of EGJ adenocarcinomas arise from long and short segments of specialized intestinal metaplasia (Barrett's esophagus). The prevalence of long segments of Barrett's esophagus (>3 cm) in patients having endoscopy for reflux symptoms is 3%, and 1% in those undergoing endoscopy for any clinical indication. However, a silent majority of patients with Barrett's esophagus remain unrecognized in the general population and may not be diagnosed unless adenocarcinoma develops. Recent studies document a rise in the diagnosis of specialized intestinal metaplasia of the cardia. Nearly all these patients have associated carditis, and *Helicobacter pylori* infection has been linked to this condition. The possible origin of EGJ adenocarcinomas in the sequence carditis – specialized intestinal metaplasia needs to be clarified. Smoking and obesity are additional risk factors for adenocarcinoma of the esophagus and EGJ. Current data does not confirm *H. pylori* as a risk factor for cancer of the EGJ.

Introduction

Cancer of the esophagus (predominantly squamous cell carcinoma) ranks among the ten most frequent cancers in the world (over 300,000 new cases per year), with most occurring in developing countries and with marked regional variations in incidence [1]. Squamous cell carcinoma is very prevalent in three regions: the Asian belt (starting in eastern Turkey and extending through the southern states of the former Soviet Union, Iran, and Iraq into northern China), parts of southern and eastern Africa, and northwestern

Recent Results in Cancer Research, Vol. 155

France. Esophageal cancer occurs much more frequently among men, and rates are typically two- to fourfold higher among men than women. However, in high-rate areas, the cancers appears almost as often in women as men, reflecting the exposure to the same causative factors [2].

The major causes of squamous cell carcinoma of the esophagus in the United States and other western countries are cigarette smoking and alcohol consumption. They have been found to be independent risk factors, and their combined effects are approximately multiplicative [3]. In the areas of the world with the very highest rates of esophageal cancer, tobacco appears not to play a major role. In these areas, dietary habits and other environmental factors seem more relevant [2].

Until 10 years ago, epidemiological studies of esophageal cancer were only focused on the most frequent histological variety, namely squamous cell carcinoma. However, the rising incidence of adenocarcinomas of the esophagus and esophagogastric junction (EGJ) in the United States and Western Europe in recent years has promoted a great deal of studies trying to explain this alarming increase in incidence and to identify possible causative factors for these adenocarcinomas [4, 5].

This review focuses on the epidemiology of adenocarcinoma of the esophagus and esophagogastric junction, describing recent trends in incidence and summarizing what is known about Barrett's esophagus as a precancerous lesion for these tumors and the role of other risk factors possibly associated with the recent increasing incidence of these carcinomas in the western world.

Rising Incidence of Adenocarcinoma of the Esophagus and Esophagogastric Junction

From 1926 to 1976, surgical series reported that adenocarcinoma of the esophagus was uncommon, representing only 0.8%–3.7% of esophageal cancers [6–9]. In recent surgical series from major referral institutions, 60%–80% of patients were diagnosed as having adenocarcinoma of the distal esophagus or EGJ compared with only 10%–15% a decade ago [10–13]. Heitmiller and colleagues [14], using the Johns Hopkins tumor registry data covering four decades (1959–1994), found that the number of new cases of adenocarcinoma of the esophagus increased sharply after 1978 and in 1994, for the first time since 1959, the number of patients with adenocarcinoma exceeded that of patients with squamous cell carcinoma (Fig. 1). The changes in the annual frequency of esophageal squamous cell carcinoma and adenocarcinoma reported in surgical series appear to be representative of what is being observed in different epidemiological studies. Population-based studies from United States and Western Europe confirm the rising incidence of adenocarcinoma of the esophagus and EGJ [4, 5, 15–18]. Data from the National Cancer Institute (NCI)'s Surveillance, Epidemiology and End Results (SEER) program, which covers nine population-based cancer registries in the United States accounting for approximately 10% of the U.S. population, indicated

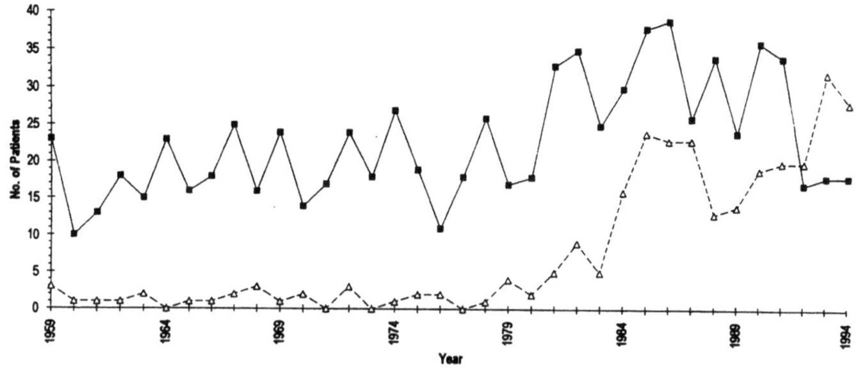

Fig. 1 Total number of patients with esophageal squamous cell carcinoma (*black squares*) and adenocarcinoma (*white triangles*) by year. (From [14] with permission)

that the incidence of esophageal adenocarcinoma in white males has doubled from the early 1970s to the late 1980s [15]. Blot and associates [4] showed that the increases in rates of esophageal adenocarcinoma in the United States through the 1980s have been on the order of 5%–10% per year, a faster pace than virtually any other cancer [16]. By 1990, adenocarcinomas accounted for nearly half of all esophageal cancers among white men [16]. Recently, Daly and colleagues [19], using the National Cancer Data Base, also confirmed the findings of other series and found a substantial increase between 1988 and 1993 in the occurrence of esophageal adenocarcinomas (from 33.2% to 43.1%). Similar trends have been seen in Denmark, the United Kingdom, Switzerland, Sweden, and Norway [5, 18, 20–22]. These observations for esophageal adenocarcinoma are paralleled by rising rates of adenocarcinoma of the EGJ [4, 24, 25]. Zheng and associates [25] examined the incidence pattern of adenocarcinoma of the EGJ and distal esophagus in Connecticut between 1955 and 1989. For males, adenocarcinoma of the EGJ increased during the study period from 0.6 per 100,000 in 1955–1959 to 3.0 per 100,000 in 1985–1989. For females, adenocarcinoma of the GEJ was low (0.1 per 100,000) and unchanged for the time period between 1955 and 1969; however, the rate increased from 0.1 per 100,000 in 1965–1969 to 0.6 per 100,000 in 1985–1989. In the West Midlands (United Kingdom), Powell and McConkey [21] found that the incidence rate of EGJ tumors increased from 0.7 to 2.0 per 100,000 between 1962 and 1981. The causes for this alarming increase in the incidence of adenocarcinomas of the esophagus and EGJ are unclear. Several risk factors for esophageal and EGJ adenocarcinomas have been proposed, as we will discuss later, including tobacco use, alcohol, dietary factors, obesity, and *Helicobacter pylori* infection. However, it is acknowledged that esophageal adenocarcinomas and a portion of EGJ adenocarcinomas arise from long or short segments of Barrett's esophagus (specialized intestinal metaplasia, SIM), a condition caused by chronic reflux of acid and duodenal contents into the esophagus.

A population-based study of adenocarcinoma, also investigating its possible association with Barrett's esophagus, has been reported in Olmsted County, Minnesota [17]. This report differs from large population studies using cancer registry data in which detailed case review is not usually performed and the histological type often remains unknown. The annual incidence of adenocarcinoma of the esophagus rose from 0.13 per 100,000 person-years in 1935–1971 to 0.74 cases per 100,000 person-years in 1974–1989. Likewise, the incidence of adenocarcinoma of the esophagogastric junction rose from 0.25 to 1.34 per 100,000 person-years when the same two periods were compared (Fig. 2). This was greater than fivefold for both cancer locations. Barrett's esophagus was found in five of eight patients (63%) with esophageal adenocarcinomas and in five of 14(36%) patients with EGJ adenocarcinomas between 1974 and 1989. In six of ten cases, Barrett's esophagus was first recognized on review of previous histological slides or new sections from preserved surgical specimens.

Distribution According to Age, Sex, and Race

Adenocarcinoma of the esophagus and EGJ show similar epidemiologic characteristics that clearly distinguish them from squamous cell carcinomas of the esophagus and from adenocarcinomas of more distal parts of the stomach. These features include very high male-to-female ratios (approximately 7:1) and a higher incidence among whites than blacks [4, 26–28]. Yang and Davis [15] found that the incidence of adenocarcinoma of the esophagus in the black population was 30% that of the white population. Zheng and colleagues [25] reported that the male to female ratio of age-adjusted incidence rates in Connecticut is approximately 5.5 for adenocarcinoma of the EGJ and

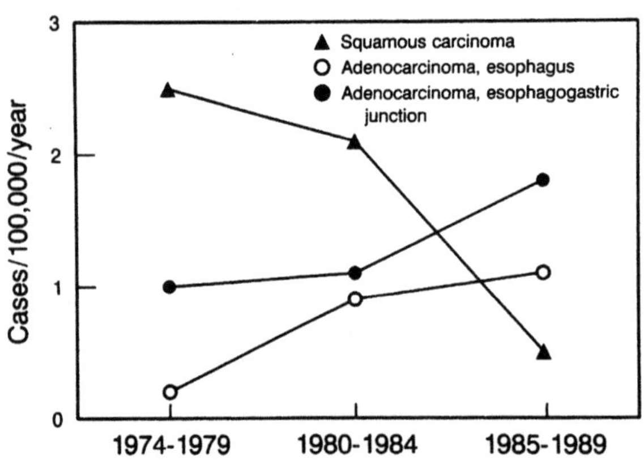

Fig. 2. Changing incidence of different types of cancer in Olmsted County from 1974 to 1989. *Triangles*, squamous carcinoma; *white circles*, adenocarcinoma of the esophagus; *black circles*, adenocarcinoma of the esophagogastric junction. (From [17] with permission)

approximately 2.2 for adenocarcinoma of the distal stomach. The white to black ratio for adenocarcinoma of the EGJ has been increasing, mainly due to a more rapid increase in the incidence of adenocarcinoma of the EGJ in whites [25]. The disease, either in the distal esophagus or at the EGJ, mostly affects patients over 50 years of age, with the peak at around 55–65 years [15].

Gastroesophageal Reflux Disease and Adenocarcinoma of the Esophagus and Esophagogastric Junction

Chow and associates [29] compared 196 patients with adenocarcinoma of the esophagus or cardia with 196 matched controls. Significant twofold or greater risks of adenocarcinoma in both locations were associated with a past history of esophageal reflux, hiatal hernia, esophagitis/ulcer, or dysphagia. The odds ratio increased with increasing number of these conditions. The cancer risk to the individual with gastroesophageal reflux disease (GERD) is small, however, because GERD is so common. Barrett's esophagus is the probable intermediate stage between GERD and adenocarcinoma [30].

Barrett's Esophagus and Adenocarcinoma of the Esophagus and Esophagogastric Junction

Barrett's esophagus is associated with GERD. In this condition, the squamous epithelium that normally lines the distal esophagus is replaced by a metaplastic columnar epithelium [31]. The intestinal-type epithelium or SIM containing goblet cells is the most common phenotype and the one which carries the risk of malignant transformation [32]. Either long (>3 cm) or short (<3 cm) segments of SIM may lead to the development of esophageal adenocarcinomas [33, 34]. Endoscopically apparent short segments of Barrett's esophagus(<3 cm) should be distinguished from SIM at the EGJ. The latter condition, increasingly recognized in recent endoscopic series, is defined as the presence of SIM below a normal-appearing squamocolumnar junction [35]. Both Barrett's esophagus and SIM at the EGJ have been implicated as possible precursor lesions for adenocarcinoma of the EGJ.

Prevalence of Barrett's Esophagus in Patients Having Endoscopy

Recent prospective endoscopic studies have found that about 3% of patients (male and female) with frequent reflux symptoms have long segments of Barrett's esophagus (LSBE) [36–38]. The inclusion of some patients with columnar-lining epithelium but without SIM in former series [39, 40] may explain their higher prevalence rates (11%–13%) of LSBE in comparison with recent series which only included patients with SIM [30]. The prevalence of LSBE in patients having endoscopy for any clinical indication is about 1% [41, 42]. The observed prevalence of short segments of Barrett's esophagus (SSBE) in unselected patients undergoing routine endoscopy is 7%–12% [43]. Others have reported SSBE in 9%–13% of patients with reflux symptoms [37, 38]. The correlation between endoscopic identification of short segments of columnar-lined esophagus and histologic evidence of SIM has been poor. In several studies, biopsy confirmed SIM in only 19%–63% of patients when endoscopy suggested SSBE [38, 44]. A recent study found that the further red mucosa extended into the lower esophagus, the higher the frequency of SIM was [45]. The increase diagnosis of SSBE in recent endoscopic series might reflect either a true increase in occurrence or an increase in the awareness and recognition of this entity, mainly instigated by its clinical importance as a precursor of esophageal and EGJ adenocarcinoma [34, 46, 47].

Prevalence of Barrett's Esophagus in the General Population

Autopsy data from Olmsted County (Minnesota) suggest that the majority of patients with Barrett's esophagus go undetected in the general population. Cameron and associates [48] found an age- and sex-adjusted prevalence of 22.6 cases per 100,000 population based on endoscopically diagnosed patients. However, the prevalence estimated by autopsy was 376 per 100,000, about 17 times more than the clinically diagnosed prevalence. These data do not take into consideration the prevalence of patients with SSBE. Cameron estimates that there are about one million individuals with Barrett's esophagus in the United States [49]. Most of them (a "silent" majority) do not know they have the condition and may not be diagnosed unless complications such as adenocarcinoma develop. Series of patients with esophageal adenocarcinomas showed that less than 10% of them were known to have had Barrett's esophagus before seeking medical attention initially because of symptoms of esophageal cancer [50]. The lack of gastroesophageal symptoms in patients with Barrett's esophagus may in part contribute to this observation [51]. Consequently, surveillance of patients known to have Barrett's esophagus for early cancer detection and treatment has only minimal impact on the population death rate from esophageal adenocarcinoma [30].

Incidence of Adenocarcinoma in Patients with Barrett's Esophagus

Follow-up studies of patients with Barrett's esophagus but not detectable neoplasm at the time of initial presentation provide information about the risk of malignant degeneration in the individual patient. In several retrospective and prospective studies of patients with LSBE, the incidence of adenocarcinoma arising in the SIM ranged from 1 in 52 to 1 in 441 patient-years of observation, with a median of about 1 in 100 patient-years of follow-up [52]. Recently, Drewith and associates [53] prospectively determined the incidence of adenocarcinoma in 177 patients with BE during a mean follow-up period of 4.8 years. Adenocarcinoma developed in four patients, an incidence of 1 in 208 patients-years of follow-up. Interestingly, the mean follow-up interval for the development of cancer was 27 months, and all patients had been diagnosed with dysplasia before they were diagnosed of cancer. The estimated risk of developing an adenocarcinoma in these studies was 30–125 times greater than in the general population [54–56]. Despite their increase risk of adenocarcinoma, most patients with Barrett's esophagus die of other causes [57].

There is no adequate information regarding the cancer risk in patients with SSBE. In a recent publication, Sharma et al. [58] prospectively determined the incidence of dysplasia in 32 patients with SSBE over a period of 36 months. The mean length was 1.5 cm. Five of these patients developed dysplasia on follow-up, three with low-grade dysplasia and two with high-grade dysplasia, the incidence of any dysplasia being 5.7% per year. One patient with high-grade dysplasia progressed to adenocarcinoma.

Prevalence of Barrett's Esophagus in Patients with Adenocarcinoma of the Esophagus and Esophagogastric Junction

Histopathological reports clearly indicate that most adenocarcinomas of the esophagus arise from columnar-lined epithelium containing SIM [33, 59]. Barrett's esophagus, like esophageal adenocarcinoma, is also much more common among men than women and among whites than blacks. EGJ adenocarcinoma has also been reported in association with Barrett's esophagus [33, 60]. Cameron and colleagues [46] found Barrett's esophagus in eight of nine patients (89%) with esophageal adenocarcinomas, the other patients having microscopic evidence of SIM. They also found Barrett's esophagus in five of 24 patients (21%) with junction adenocarcinoma, five more having microscopic evidence of SIM involving less than 3 cm. Smaller junction tumors (<6 cm) were more often associated with SIM than larger tumors. These authors suggested that many, perhaps most, junction cancers arise in a short or long segment of SIM, but the enlarging cancer may grow over and conceal the underlying Barrett's epithelium in which it arose. Clark and associates [47] found histologic evidence of SIM in 42% of adenocarcinomas of the EGJ and in 79% of esophageal adenocarcinomas. The length of Barrett's mucosa associated with EGJ tumors was shorter than that found in the esophageal tumors, and Barrett's esophagus was therefore frequently missed during preoperative endoscopy and biopsy.

Possible Relationship Between Adenocarcinomas of the Esophagogastric Junction and Specialized Intestinal Metaplasia at the Esophagogastric Junction

It has been suggested that EGJ adenocarcinomas might have two possible origins: either from areas of SIM in the distal esophagus (Barrett's esophagus) or from multifocal areas of atrophic gastritis and intestinal metaplasia at the cardia, below a normal squamocolumnar junction [61]. Recent studies document a rise in the diagnosis of SIM at the EGJ. The observed prevalence of SIM below a normal-appearing squamous–columnar junction was 5%–23% in several series of patients having endoscopy for a variety of upper gastrointestinal symptoms [41–44, 62]. Cameron and colleagues [37, 38] found SIM at the EGJ in 8%–14% of patients with reflux symptoms. Of interest, SIM at the EGJ was also found in 25% of controls. Nearly all patients with intestinal metaplasia of the cardia have associated carditis [61]. Current data do not support the hypothesis that carditis is an inflammatory change that occurs as a consequence of GERD [61]. It is possible that, unlike in traditional Barrett's esophagus, in which acid reflux is the most important factor for the development of intestinal metaplasia, the inflammation at the EGJ due to other causes is the initiating factor. It seems that *H. pylori* infection might be the cause of most cases of inflammation and associated SIM at the EGJ [63, 64]. At present, the possible role of intestinal metaplasia at the EGJ as a premalignant lesion for EGJ adenocarcinomas is not yet clear. The importance of confirming this relationship lies in the potential benefit of surveillance endoscopy in all patients with this histologic diagnosis. However, it is likely that, if SIM is so common, then the cancer risk and usefulness of surveillance biopsies for an individual patient would be low. The possible origin of EGJ adenocarcinomas from the sequence carditis – atrophic gastritis – intestinal metaplasia – dysplasia needs to be clarified. The identification of multiple environmental factors probably acting synergistically to induce malignant transformation in this sequence will be the next step toward identifying the population at risk for adenocarcinoma of the EGJ.

Additional Risk Factors for Adenocarcinoma of the Esophagus and Esophagogastric Junction

Except for Barrett's esophagus, little is known about other factors involved in the etiology of these adenocarcinomas. The risk factors that have been proposed for esophageal and esophagogastric junction adenocarcinomas include smoking, alcohol, obesity, dietary factors, and *H. pylori* infection.

Smoking, Alcohol, Obesity, and Diet

Smoking and drinking have been found to be more prevalent in patients with adenocarcinoma of the esophagus than in those with uncomplicated Barrett's esophagus in some but not all reports [65–67].

A recent large-scale case-control study has added definitive evidence on the effect of smoking on the risk of esophageal and EGJ adenocarcinomas [68]. Risk appears to be more than doubled, with a dose–response pattern among smokers. Little reduction in risk was observed until smoking cessation for more than 30 years, which is in contrast to the steady decrease in risk observed after quitting for other smoking-related cancers such as cancer of the lung and squamous cell carcinoma of the esophagus. Gammon and colleagues [68] suggest that smoking may affect an early stage in the induction of esophageal and EGJ adenocarcinomas, whereas later stages are involved for esophageal squamous cell carcinoma. Although these data support the role of tobacco as an etiologic factor in adenocarcinomas of the esophagus and EGJ, it does not explain the rising incidence of these adenocarcinomas at a time when squamous cell carcinoma of the esophagus is not increasing and there have been recent reductions in the prevalence of cigarette smoking [69].

A recent multicenter population-based, case-control study revealed that excess weight is a strong risk factor for esophageal adenocarcinoma, with risk rising with increasing body mass index (BMI) [70]. To a lesser extent, excess weight increased the risk of esophagogastric junction adenocarcinomas, while no effect was seen for gastric adenocarcinoma or esophageal squamous cell carcinoma. The positive association between risk of esophageal adenocarcinoma and usual BMI was significantly modified by age, with the greatest increase in risk seen among the youngest group (<50 years). This finding suggests that obesity is a particularly important factor in early-onset tumors, while other risk factors may assume a more prominent role in tumors developing in later years. The mechanism by which excess weight might affect the risk of adenocarcinoma of the esophagus and EGJ is not clear. One hypothesis suggests that, by increasing the risk of hiatal hernia and GERD, obesity would presumably increase the risk of Barrett's esophagus, which in turn is a precursor lesion for esophageal adenocarcinoma [71]. Additional factors that may influence the cancer risks associated with obesity and GERD, including body fat distribution, dietary practices, medications, and other conditions that may affect the composition of the enterogastric refluxate, should be investigated in the near future [70].

A recent case-control study identified high intake of dietary calories and fat as risk factors for adenocarcinoma [72]. In addition, an inverse association between fruit and vegetable consumption and esophageal and EGJ adenocarcinoma has been shown [71]. These studies suggest that the risk of adenocarcinoma of the esophagus and EGJ might be reduced in the near future through dietary interventions.

Helicobacter pylori Infection

There is strong evidence for *H. pylori* infection as a cause of chronic atrophic gastritis and intestinal metaplasia, two possible precancerous lesions for gastric cancer. The results of a recent meta-analysis have quantitatively confirmed that *H. pylori* is an important risk factor in gastric cancer but not in cancer of the cardia [73]. The risk of gastric adenocarcinoma and its precursor state, atrophic gastritis, is particularly associated with *cagA*$^+$ compared with *cagA*$^-$ strains of *H. pylori* [74]. Of interest, a recent study found an inverse relation between *cagA*$^+$ strains of *H. pylori* infection and risk of esophageal and gastric cardia adenocarcinoma [75]. The reduced risk of adenocarcinomas of the esophagus and gastric cardia associated with *cagA*$^+$ infection is consistent with recent clinical reports that *cagA*$^-$ strains predominate among patients with esophageal adenocarcinoma and the precursor states of gastroesophageal reflux disease, Barrett's esophagus and esophageal dysplasia [76, 77]. It will be of interest to evaluate whether variations in acidity and content of refluxate are involved in the mechanism by which *H. pylori* strains may affect the risk of adenocarcinoma of the esophagus and esophagogastric junction [75].

Genetic Factors

Familial occurrence of Barrett's esophagus and esophageal adenocarcinoma, occurring in successive generations, has been reported [78–80]. An autosomal dominant inheritance for Barrett's esophagus has been proposed in some families [80, 81]. However, it remains unclear whether genetic abnormalities directly predispose individuals to columnar metaplasia or result in a propensity to GERD with Barrett's esophagus and adenocarcinoma occurring as late complications of reflux-induced esophageal mucosal damage. Recently, Romero and associates [82] found that reflux symptoms were significantly more prevalent among parents and siblings of patients with adenocarcinoma (43% vs. 23%) and Barrett's esophagus (46% vs. 27%) than spouse control relatives. No significant difference was found for the reflux esophagitis group (33% vs. 29%). They concluded that there may be a genetic predisposition to the development of reflux in families with Barrett's esophagus and esophageal adenocarcinoma. They also noted a major trend of high GERD prevalence rates in the adult children of probands with Barrett's esophagus and adenocarcinoma, suggesting that the predisposition to GERD may be passed on to the next generation.

Acknowledgements. The author thanks Dr. Luis Grande for his help during the preparation of this manuscript.

References

1. Parkin DM, Pisani P, Ferlay J (1993) Estimates of the worldwide incidence of eighteen major cancers in 1985. Int J Cancer 54:1–13
2. Blot WJ (1994) Esophageal cancer trends and risk factors. Semin Oncol 21:403–410
3. Tuyns AJ, Pèquignot G, Jensen OM (1977) Le cancer de l'oesophage en Ille-et-Vilaine en fonction des niveaux de consommation d'alcohol et de tabac. Des risques qui se multiplient. Bull Cancer 64:45–60
4. Blot WJ, Devesa SS, Kneller RW, Fraumeni JF (1991) Rising incidence of adenocarcinoma of the esophagus and gastric cardia. JAMA 265:1287–1289
5. Reed PI, Johnston BJ (1993) The changing incidence of oesophageal cancer. Endoscopy 25:606–608
6. Bosch A, Frias Z, Caldwell WL (1979) Adenocarcinoma of the esophagus. Cancer 43:1557–1561
7. Puestow CB, Gillesby WJ, Guynn VL (1955) Cancer of the esophagus. Arch Surg 70:662–668
8. Turnbull ADM, Goodner JT (1968) Primary adenocarcinoma of the esophagus. Cancer 22:915–918
9. Webb JN, Busuttil A (1978) Adenocarcinoma of the esophagus and of the oesophagogastric junction. Br J Surg 65:475–479
10. Gelfand GEJ, Finley RJ, Nelems B (1992) Transhiatal esophagectomy for carcinoma of the esophagus and cardia. Arch Surg 127:1164–1167
11. Putnam JB, Suell DM, McMurtrey M (1994) Comparison of three techniques of esophagectomy within a residency training program. Ann Thorac Surg 57:319–325
12. Millikan KW, Silverstein J, Hart V, Blair K, Bines S, Roberts J, Doolas A (1995) A 15-year review of esophagectomy for carcinoma of the esophagus and cardia. Arch Surg 130:617–624
13. Rice TW, Zuccaro G, Adelstein DJ, Rybicki LA, Blackstone EH, Goldblum JR (1998) Esophageal carcinoma: depth of tumor invasion is predictive of regional lymph node status. Ann Thorac Surg 65:787–792
14. Heitmiller RF, Sharma RR (1996) Comparison of prevalence and resection rates in patients with esophageal squamous cell carcinoma and adenocarcinoma. J Thorac Cardiovasc Surg 112:130–136
15. Yang PC, Davis S (1988) Incidence of cancer of the esophagus in the US by histologic type. Cancer 61:612–617
16. Blot WJ, Devesa SS, Fraumeni JF (1993) Continuing climb in rates of esophageal adenocarcinoma: an update (letter). JAMA 270:1320
17. Pera M, Cameron AJ, Trastek VF, Carpenter HA, Zinsmeister AR (1993) Increasing incidence of adenocarcinoma of the esophagus and esophagogastric junction. Gastroenterology 104:510–513
18. Hansson LE, Sparen P, Nyren O (1993) Increasing incidence of both major histological types of esophageal carcinomas among men in Sweden. Int J Cancer 54:402–407
19. Daly JM, Karnell LH, Menck HR (1996) National Cancer Data Base Report on esophageal carcinoma. Cancer 78:1820–1828
20. Moller H (1992) Incidence of cancer of the esophagus, cardia and stomach in Denmark. Eur J Cancer Prev 1:159–164
21. Powell J, McConkey CC (1990) Increasing incidence of adenocarcinoma of the gastric cardia and adjacent sites. Br J Cancer 62:440–443
22. Levi F, LaVecchia C (1991) Adenocarcinoma of the esophagus in Switzerland (letter). JAMA 265:2960
23. Hansen S, Wiig JN, Giercksky KE, Tretli S (1997) Esophageal and gastric carcinoma in Norway 1958–1992: incidence time trend variability according to morphological subtypes and organ subsites. Int J Cancer 71:340–344
24. Powell J, McConkey CC (1992) The rising trend in esophageal adenocarcinoma and gastric cardia. Eur J Cancer Prev 1:265–269

25. Zheng T, Mayne ST, Holford TR, Boyle P, Liu W, Chen Y, Mador M, Flannery J (1993) The time trend and age-period-cohort effects on incidence of adenocarcinoma of the stomach in Connecticut from 1955–1989. Cancer 72:330–340
26. Kalish RJ, Clancy PE, Orringer MB, Appleman HD (1984) Clinical epidemiologic and morphologic comparison between adenocarcinomas arising in Barrett's esophageal mucosa and gastric cardia. Gastroenterology 86:461–467
27. Rogers EL, Goldkind SF, Iseri OA, Bustin, M, Goldkin, L, Hamilton, SR, Smith, RRL (1986) Adenocarcinoma of the lower esophagus. A disease primarily of white men with Barrett's esophagus. J Clin Gastroenterol 8:613–618
28. Wang HH, Antonioli DA, Goldman H (1986) Comparative features of esophageal and gastric adenocarcinomas: recent changes in type and frequency. Hum Pathol 17:482–487
29. Chow WH, Finkle WD, McLaughin JK, Frankl H, Ziel HZ, Fraumeni JF (1995) The relation of gastroesophageal reflux disease and its treatment to adenocarcinoma of the esophagus and gastric cardia. JAMA 274:474–477
30. Cameron AJ (1997) Epidemiology of columnar-lined esophagus and adenocarcinoma. Gastroenterol Clin North Am 26:487–494
31. Spechler SJ, Goyal RK (1996) The columnar-lined esophagus, intestinal metaplasia, and Norman Barrett. Gastroenterology 110:614–621
32. Weinstein WM, Ippoliti AF (1996) The diagnosis of Barrett's esophagus: goblets, goblets, goblets. Gastrointest Endosc 44:91–95
33. Hamilton SR, Smith RR (1987) The relationship between columnar epithelial dysplasia and invasive adenocarcinoma arising in Barrett's esophagus. Am J Clin Pathol 87:301–312
34. Schnell TG, Sontag SJ, Chejfec G (1992) Adenocarcinoma arising in tongues or short segments of Barrett's esophagus. Dig Dis Sci 37:137–143
35. Spechler SJ (1997) Short and ultrashort Barrett's esophagus – what does it mean? Semin Gastrointest Dis 8:59–67
36. Abo SR, Stevens M, Abedi PHR, Green GJ, Lightdale H, Bezwada H, Rotterdam H, Garcia-Carrasquillo RJ, Siegel LM (1995) Prevalence of short-segment Barrett's epithelium in patients with gastroesophageal reflux diasease (abstract). Gastroenterology 108:A43
37. Cameron AJ, Kamath PS, Carpenter HC (1995) Barrett's esophagus: the prevalence of short and long segments in reflux patients (abstract). Gastroenterology 108:A65
38. Cameron AJ, Kamath PS, Carpenter HC (1997) Prevalence of Barrett's esophagus and intestinal metaplasia at the esophagogastric junction (abstract). Gastroenterology 112:A82
39. Mann NS, Tsai MF, Nair PK (1989) Barrett's esophagus in patients with symptomatic reflux esophagitis. Am J Gastroenterol 84:1494–1496
40. Winters C, Spurling TJ, Chobanian SJ, Curtis DJ, Esposito RL, Hacker JF, Johnson DA, Cruess DF, Cotelingan JD, Gurney MS, Cattau EL (1987) Barrett's esophagus: a prevalent, occult complication of gastroesophageal reflux disease. Gastroenterology 92:118–124
41. Spechler SJ, Zeroogian JM, Antonioli DA, Wang HH, Goyal RK (1994) Prevalence of metaplasia at the gastro-oesophageal junction. Lancet 344:1533–1336
42. Johnston MH, Hammond AS, Laskin H, Jones DM (1996) The prevalence and clinical characteristics of short segments of specialized intestinal metaplasia in the distal esophagus on routine endoscopy. Am J Gastroenterol 91:1507–1511
43. Hirota WK, Loughney TM, Lazas DJ, Maydonovich CL, Rhol V, Wong RKH (1997) The prevalence and demographics of specialized intestinal metaplasia at the esophagogastric junction in a cohort of 889 prospectively studied patients (abstract). Gastroenterology 112:A149
44. Morales TG, Sampliner RE, Bhattacharyya T (1997) Intestinal metaplasia of the cardia. Am J Gastroenterol 92:444–418
45. Dias-Pereira A, Suspiro A, Chaves P, Saraiva A, Glória L, Mendes de Almeida JC, Leitao CN, Soares J, Mira FC (1998) Short segments of Barrett's epithelium and intestinal me-

taplasia in normal appearing oesophagogastric junctions: the same or two different entities? Gut 42:659–662
46. Cameron AJ, Lomboy CT, Pera M, Carpenter HA (1995) Adenocarcinoma of the esophagogastric junction and Barrett's esophagus. Gastroenterology 109:1541–1546
47. Clark GWB, Smyrk TC, Burdiles P, Hoef SF, Peter, JH, Kiyab, M, Hinder RA, Bremner CG, DeMeester TR (1994) Is Barrett's metaplasia the source of adenocarcinomas of the cardia? Arch Surg 129:609–614
48. Cameron AJ, Zinsmeister AR, Ballard DJ, Carney JA (1990) Prevalence of columnar-lined (Barrett's) esophagus: comparison of population-based clinical and autopsy findings. Gastroenterology 99:918–922
49. Cameron AJ (1993) Epidemiologic studies and the development of Barrett's esophagus. Endoscopy 25:635–636
50. Menke-Pluymers MB, Schoute NW, Mulder AH, Hop WC, van Blankenstein M, Tilanus HW (1992) Outcome of surgical treatment of adenocarcinoma in Barrett's esophagus. Gut 33:1454–1458
51. GOSPE (1991) Barrett's esophagus: epidemiological and clinical results of a multicentric survey. Int J Cancer 48:364–368
52. Tytgat GNJ (1995) Does endoscopic surveillance in esophageal columnar metaplasia (Barrett's esophagus) have any real value? Endoscopy 27:19–26
53. Drewitz DJ, Sampliner RE, Garewal HS (1997) The incidence of adenocarcinoma in Barrett's esophagus: a prospective study of 170 patients followed 4.8 years. Am J Gastroenterol 92:212–215
54. Cameron AJ, Ott BJ, Payne WS (1985) The incidence of adenocarcinoma in columnar-lined (Barrett's esophagus). N Engl J Med 131:857–859
55. Hameeteman W, Tytgat GNJ, Houthoff HJ, Van Den Theel JG (1989) Barrett's esophagus: development of dysplasia and adenocarcinoma. Gastroenterology 96:1249–1256
56. Robertson CS, Mayberry JR, Nicholson DA, James PD, Atkinson M (1988) Value of endoscopic surveillance in the detection of neoplastic change in Barrett's esophagus. Br J Surg 75:760–763
57. Van der Burgh A, Dees J, Hop WCJ, van Blankenstein M (1996) Oesophageal cancer is an uncommon cause of death in patients with Barrett's esophagus. Gut 39:5–8
58. Sharma P, Morales T, Bhattacharyya A, Garewal HS, Sampliner RE (1997) Dysplasia in short-segment Barrett's esophagus: a prospective 3-year follow-up. Am J Gastroenterol 92:2012–2016
59. Haggitt RC, Tryzelaar J, Ellis FH, Colcher H (1978) Adenocarcinoma complicating columnar epithelium-lined (Barrett's) esophagus. Am J Clin Pathol 70:1–5
60. Thompson JJ, Zeinsser KR, Enterline HT (1983) Barrett's metaplasia an adenocarcinoma of the esophagus and gastroesophageal junction. Hum Pathol 14:42–60
61. Richter JE (1998) Intestinal metaplasia and the squamocolumnar junction: what does it all mean? Gut 42:604–605
62. Chalasani N, Wo JM, Hunter JG, Waring JP (1997) Significance of intestinal metaplasia in different areas of esophagus including esophagogastric junction. Dig Dis Sci 42:603–607
63. Hirota WK, Loughney TM, Lazas DJ, Maydonovich CL, Rhol V, Wong RKH (1997) Is Helicobacter pylori associated with specialized intestinal metaplasia of the esophagus or stomach? A prospective study of 889 patients (abstract). Gastroenterology 112:A149
64. Peek RM, Vaezi MF, Goldblum JR, Falk GW, Vicari JJ, Perez-Perez GI, Rice TW, Sechopoulos P, Richter JE, Blaser MJ (1998) Seropositivity to *CagA*, HspA, and IgA identifies *Helicobacter pylori* strains that induce premalignant changes in the gastric cardia but not in the esophagus (abstract). Gastroenterology 114:A661
65. Gray MR, Kingsnorth AN (1990) The role of smoking and alcohol in metaplasia and cancer risk in Barrett's columnar lined esophagus. Gut 34:727–731
66. Menke-Pluymers MBE, Hop WC, Dees J, van Blankenstein M, Tilanus HW (1993) Risk factors for the development of an adenocarcinoma in columnar-lined (Barrett's) esophagus. Cancer 72:1155–1158

67. Levi F, Ollyo JB, La Vecchia C, Boyle P, Monnier P, Savary M (1990) The consumption of tobacco, alcohol and the risk of adenocarcinoma in Barrett's esophagus. Int J Cancer 45:852–854
68. Gammon MD, Shoenberg JB, Ahsan H, Risch HA, Vaughan TL, Chow WH, Rotterdam H, West AB, Dubrow R, Stanford JL, Mayne ST, Farrow DC, Niwa S, Blot WJ, Fraumeni JF (1997) Tobacco, alcohol, and socioeconomic status and adenocarcinomas of the esophagus and gastric cardia. J Natl Cancer Inst 89:1277–1284
69. Zhang ZF, Kurtz RC, Marshall JR (1997) Cigarette smoking and esophageal and gastric cardia adenocarcinoma. J Nat Cancer Inst 89:1247–1248
70. Chow WH, Blot WJ, Vaughan TL, Risch HA, Gammon MD, Stanford JL, Dubrow R, Schoenberg JB, Mayne ST, Farrow DC, Ahsan H, West AB, Rotterdam H, Niwa S, Fraumeni JF (1998) Body mass index and risk of adenocarcinoma of the esophagus and gastric cardia. J Natl Cancer Inst 90:150–105
71. Brown LM, Swanson CA, Gridley G, Swanson GM, Schoenberg JB, Greenberg RS, Silverman DT, Pottern LM, Hayes RB, Schwarz AG, Liff JM, Fraumeni JF, Hoover RN (1995) Adenocarcinoma of the esophagus: role of obesity and diet. J Natl Cancer Inst 87:104–109
72. Zhang ZF, Kurtz RC, Yu GP, Gargon N, Karpeh M, Fein JS, Harlap S (1997) Adenocarcinomas of the esophagus and gastric cardia: the role of diet. Nutr Cancer 27:298–309
73. Huang JQ, Subbaramiah S, Chen Y, Hunt RH (1998) Meta-analysis of the relationship between *Helicobacter pylori* seropositivity and gastric cancer. Gastroenterology 114:1169–1179
74. Parsonnet J, Friedman GD, Orentreich N, Vogelman JH (1997) Risk for gastric cancer in people with *CagA* positive or *CagA* negative *Helicobacter pylori* infection. Gut 40:297–301
75. Chow WH, Blaser MJ, Blot WJ, Gammon MD, Vaughan TL, Risch HA, Perez-Perez I, Schoenberg JB, Stanford JL, Rotterdam H, West AB, Fraumeni JF (1998) An inverse relation between $cagA^{+}$ strains of *Helicobacter pylory* infection and risk of esophageal and gastric cardia adenocarcinoma. Cancer Res 58:588–590
76. Grimley CE, Loff DE, Morris AG, Nwakolo CU (1997) Virulent *Helicobacter pylori* (HP) in patients with gastric and esophageal adenocarcinoma (abstract). Gastroenterology 112:A571
77. Schnell JW, Vicari JJ, Perez-Perez GI, Falk GW, Halter SA, Goldblum JR, Gangarosa LM, Rice TW, Richter JE, Blaser MJ, Peek RM (1997) *Helicobacter pylori* $cagA^{-}$ strains predominate in gastroesophageal reflux disease, Barrett's esophagus and esophageal dysplasia/adenocarcinoma (abstract). Gastroenterology 112:A283
78. Eng C, Spechler SJ, Ruben R, Li FP (1993) Familial Barrett's esophagus and adenocarcinoma of the gastroesophageal junction. Cancer Epidemiol Biomark Prev 2:397–399
79. Crabb DW, Berk MA, Hall TR, Conneally PM, Biegel AA, Lehman GA (1985) Familial gastroesophageal reflux and development of Barrett's esophagus. Ann Intern Med 103:52–54
80. Fahmy N, King JF (1993) Barrett's esophagus: an acquired condition with genetic predisposition. Am J Gastroenterol 88:1262–1265
81. Jochen VJ, Fuerst PA, Fromkes JJ (1992) Familial Barrett's esophagus associated with adenocarcinoma. Gastroenterology 102:1400–1402
82. Romero Y, Cameron AJ, Locke R, Schaid, DJ, Slezak JM, Branch CD, Melton LJ (1997) Familial agreggation of gastroesophageal reflux in patients with Barrett's esophagus and esophageal adenocarcinoma. Gastroenterology 113:1449–1456

Modern Pathology: Prognostic Parameters in Squamous Cell Carcinoma of the Esophagus

M. Sarbia, H.E. Gabbert

Institut für Pathologie, Heinrich Heine Universität, Moorenstr. 5,
40225 Düsseldorf, Germany

Abstract

In the present study the prognostic impact of new histological and molecular parameters were tested retrospectively in a series of 149 patients with esophageal squamous cell carcinoma (SCC) who underwent potentially curative resection therapy. In addition, the prognostic value of various molecular markers was investigated in a group of 38 patients with locally advanced esophageal SCC treated using combined therapy modalities. In the surgically treated carcinomas, the following morphological parameters proved to be prognostically significant in univariate survival analysis and multivariate survival analysis: pattern of invasion, inflammatory response, and lymph vessel invasion. In contrast, tumor grading according to the criteria of the WHO and tumor cell proliferation did not show significant prognostic impact. Concerning the prognostic influence of molecular parameters, strong expression of the proliferation regulating molecule $p21^{WAF1}$ and weak expression of the apoptosis regulating molecule Bcl-X_L were predictors of poor survival in univariate and multivariate survival analysis. No prognostic impact was shown in relation to the expression of p53 and the apoptosis regulating molecules Bcl-2 and Bax. In the multimodally treated esophageal cancer patients, strong expression of $p21^{WAF1}$ and accumulation of p53 were predictors of poor survival, whereas expression of Bcl-2, Bax, and Bcl-X_L had no prognostic significance. In conclusion, morphological and molecular parameters may provide important prognostic information for esophageal cancer patients.

Introduction

Surgical resection is the standard therapy for resectable esophageal cancer, but the overall survival is still poor and considerable efforts have been made to improve the therapeutic results by new adjuvant or neoadjuvant therapeutic modalities [6, 8, 13]. In this situation, modern pathology has to deal with two basic questions: (1) whether it can help to identify those patients who

Recent Results in Cancer Research, Vol. 155

are at a higher risk and (2) whether it can help to identify those patients who may benefit from those new therapeutic modalities. In the present study, two different approaches have been followed to target these questions. First, new potential histological and molecular parameters (Table 1) were tested retrospectively in a series of 149 patients with esophageal squamous cell carcinoma (SCC) who underwent standard therapy by R0 resection (no distant metastases, no residual tumor, no radiotherapy or chemotherapy). This analysis was performed in order to identify patients with an increased risk for tumor-related death who were thus being candidates for new adjuvant therapeutic strategies in the future. Second, the prognostic value of the molecular markers was investigated in a group of 38 patients with locally advanced esophageal SCC treated with combined therapy modalities (radiochemotherapy and optionally surgery) (Fig. 1). [26]. In this analysis, it was examined whether the determination of tumor-associated molecular markers in pretherapeutic biopsies may help to predict response to therapy and overall survival of patients treated by multimodal therapy.

Morphological Parameters in Surgically Treated Esophageal Cancer Patients

Grading

Histopathologic typing, grading, and staging of resected tumors are is carried out in an attempt to predict the outcome of cancer patients. In esophageal cancer, the definitive pathologic stage according to the TNM classification of tumors [9] and the macroscopic and microscopic determination of tu-

Table 1. Prognostic parameters in esophageal cancer

Status	Parameters
Established	pT category
	pN category
	pM category
	R category
Potential	
Morphological	Grading (WHO)
	Pattern of invasion
	Inflammatory response
	Blood vessel invasion
	Lymph vessel invasion
Molecular	p53
	$p21^{WAF1}$
	Rb
	Bcl-2
	Bax
	Bcl-x_L

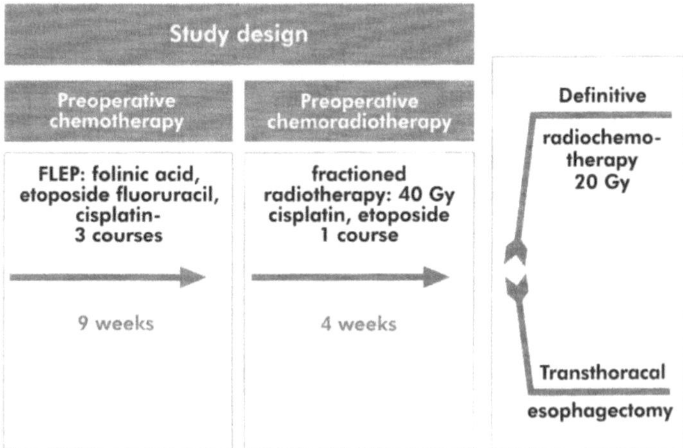

Fig. 1. Multimodal treatment of 38 patients with locally advanced squamous cell carcinoma of the esophagus

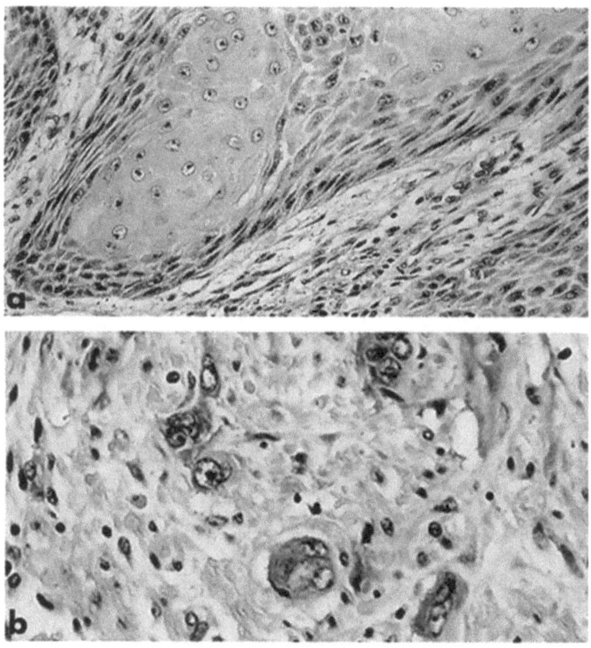

Fig. 2. Histological examples of tumors with **a** a pushing type of invasion and **b** a dissociated type of invasion

mor tissue at the resection margins (R classification) are generally accepted prognostic parameters [11, 12]. In contrast, the traditional grading systems as proposed by the World Health Organization (WHO) [31] or the Japanese Society for Esophageal Diseases [10], which are mainly based on the degree of tumor differentiation, mitotic activity, and nuclear abnormalities, have not

Table 2. Survival rates (%) of 149 surgically treated patients with SCC of the esophagus in relation to the new prognostic score and tumor differentiation. Log-rank test

Parameter	(*n*)	2-years	5-years	*p*-value
Prognostic score				0.0001
group 1	24	66.7	66.7	
group 2	35	51.4	30.8	
group 3	71	33.8	12.3	
group 4	19	21.1	5.3	
Grading				NS
G1	15	73.3	52.5	
G2	62	37.1	27.3	
G3	46	41.3	12.8	
G4	26	34.6	22.4	

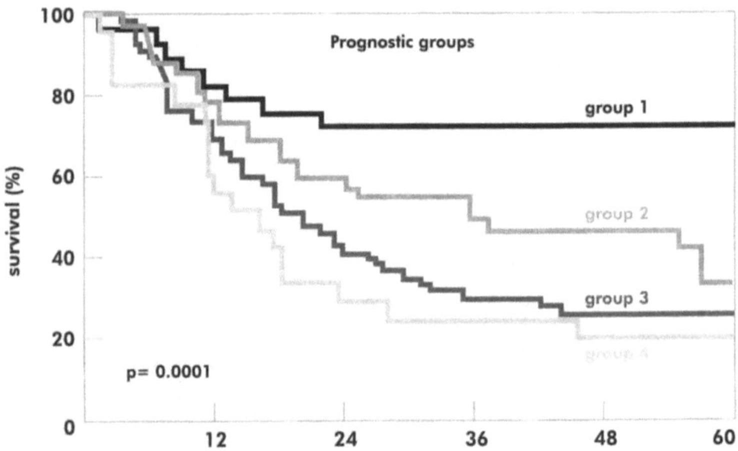

Fig. 3. Overall survival rate of 149 surgically treated esophageal cancer patients in relation to the morphologic prognostic score ($p=0.0001$; combination of the parameters inflammatory response and pattern of invasion)

proved to be prognostically significant [4, 28]. We therefore analyzed two new morphological parameters, i. e. pattern of invasion and inflammatory response of the host tissue. In summary, we were able to show that the survival rates significantly decreased when the pattern of invasion changed from a pushing cohesive pattern to a dissociated infiltrating pattern (Fig. 2) and significantly decreased when the inflammatory response of the host tissue changed from a strong to a weak or negative reaction. Putting both parameters together in a score system, four different prognostic groups were defined (Table 2). In contrast to the WHO grading, which failed to be prognostically significant, highly significant differences in survival were able to be verified between these prognostic groups by both uni- and multivariate analysis [22] (Fig. 3).

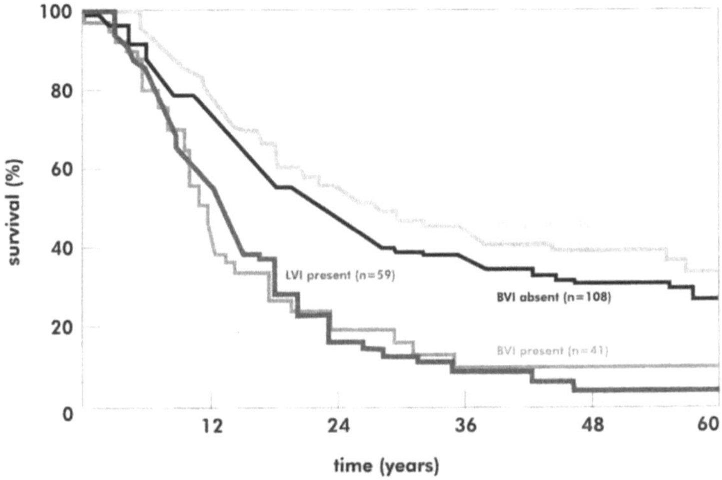

Fig. 4. Overall survival rate of 149 surgically treated esophageal cancer patients in relation to the parameters lymphatic vessel invasion (*LVI*, $p=0.0001$) and blood vessel invasion (*BVI*; $p=0.0005$)

Vascular Invasion

Vascular invasion, another morphological parameter, has already been associated with poor survival in different human malignancies such as breast cancer [16] colorectal cancer [29], and gastric cancer [7]. In our study on esophageal cancer, blood vessel invasion was detected in 27.5% and lymphatic vessel invasion in 39.6% of all patients. As shown by univariate analysis, the survival rate of patients with proven blood vessel invasion was significantly worse than that of patients without blood vessel invasion ($p=0.0005$), and the same applied to patients with lymphatic vessel invasion ($p=0.0001$) [23] (Fig. 4).

Proliferative Activity

Concerning the potential prognostic role of tumor cell proliferation, the majority of studies published so far seem to confirm a negative impact on survival in different types of cancer [1, 18], but there are also studies denying such a correlation [15]. In our own study, the monoclonal antibody MIB-1 was used, which recognizes an epitope of the Ki-67 antigen [2] and which produces a strong immunoreaction confined to the nuclei. Considering only the areas of highest proliferative activity, a median proliferation index of 34% was found. However, there was a striking heterogeneity between the different tumors, with the highest proliferation index ranging between 5% and nearly 100% (Fig. 5). With respect to survival, no differences between tumors with a proliferation index higher and lower than the median value could be verified, however,

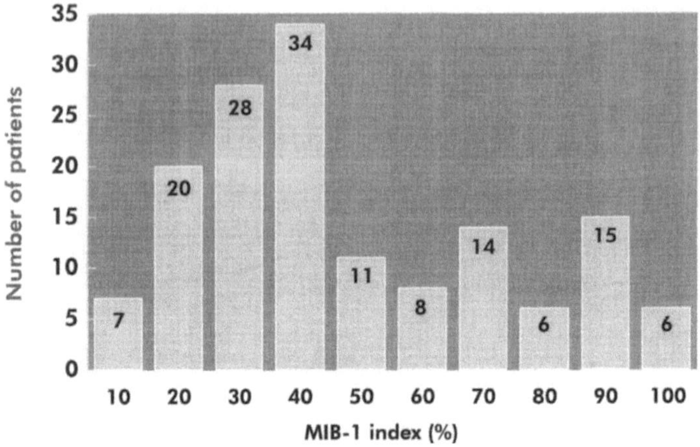

Fig. 5. Marked heterogeneity in proliferative activity among 149 squamous cell carcinomas (SCC) of the esophagus

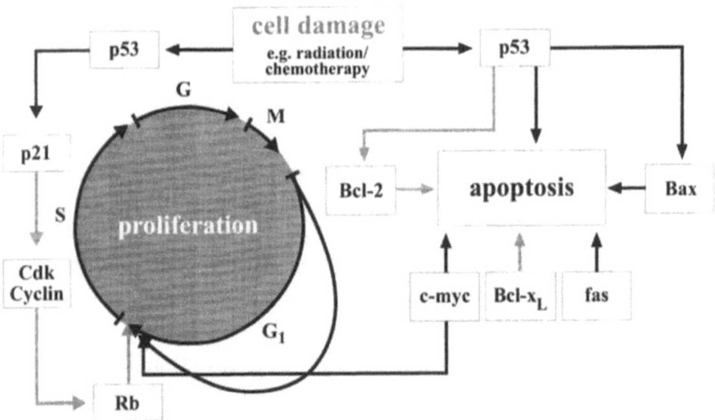

Fig. 6. Simplified scheme of molecules involved in the regulation of proliferation and apoptosis. *Black paths*, activating; *gray paths*, inhibiting

and this also held true when different cut off points ranging from 10% to 90% proliferation indices were calculated or when different subgroups of patients (e.g., nodal-negative patients) were considered separately [24].

Multivariate Survival Analysis of the Morphological Candidates

Comparing the morphological prognostic parameters under investigation with the prognostic value of the established pTNM system by means of a multivariate Cox regression analysis, only the parameters lymph vessel invasion (LVI; $p=0.0001$), the new prognostic score system ($p=0.0015$), and the pN category ($p=0.0095$) maintained their prognostic significance.

Molecular Parameters in Surgically Treated Esophageal Cancer Patients

Our investigation on the prognostic role of molecular parameters in esophageal cancer focused on proteins that are part of the signaling network regulating proliferation and apoptosis. These genes may not only be important for the growth of esophageal cancers, but to our current knowledge also substantially influence the efficacy of radiotherapy and/or chemotherapy (Fig. 6).

p 53

In the regulation of proliferation and apoptosis, the tumor suppressor gene p 53 is a crucial molecule giving a damaged tumor cell two options: either to stop proliferation with a chance for repair or, if the damage is too severe, to commit suicide through apoptosis [17]. In our own immunohistochemical investigation, we used the monoclonal antibody DO-1 (Oncogene Science), which recognizes wild-type and mutant p 53 and gives a distinct muclear staining reaction. p 53 expression was found in 65.1% of all carcinomas, but there was a striking heterogeneity between different tumors, with only a very low p 53 expression in many tumors. No correlations were found between p 53 expression and other parameters such as pT and pN category or grading. With regard to survival, no differences between p 53-positive and p 53-negative patients were found (Fig. 7), and this was also true when different levels of p 53 expression or different subgroups of patients were considered [21].

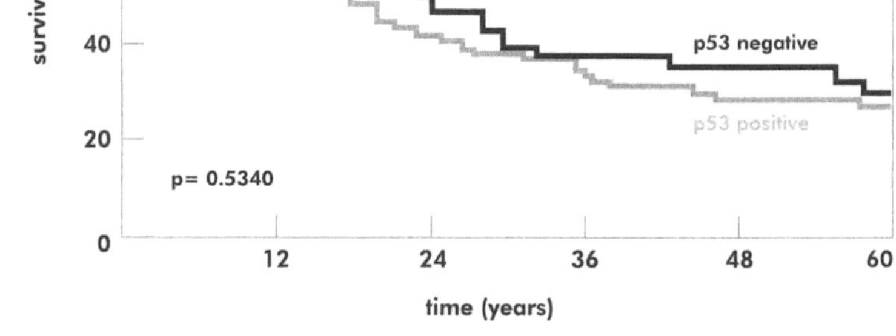

Fig. 7. Overall survival of 149 surgically treated esophageal cancer patients in relation to p 53 expression in the tumor tissue

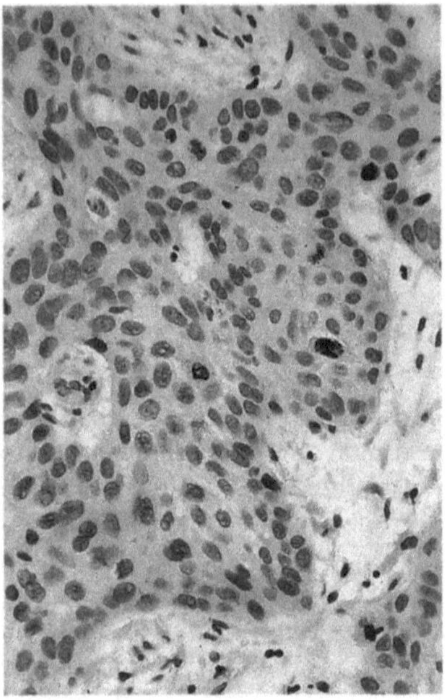

Fig. 8. Immunohistochemical detection of p21^{WAF1} expression in the nuclei of a moderately differentiated squamous cell carcinoma (SCC) of the esophagus

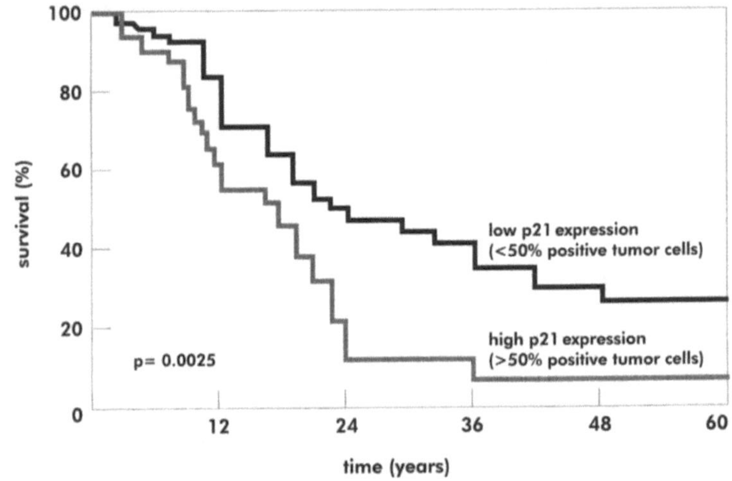

Fig. 9. Overall survival of 149 surgically treated esophageal cancer patients in relation to p21^{WAF1} expression in the tumor tissue ($p=0.0025$)

p21^{WAF1}

Closely related to p53 is p21^{WAF1} (wild-type p53-activated fragment 1), which inhibits proliferation by inhibiting cyclin-dependent kinases [5]. Located in the tumor cell nuclei (Fig. 8), its overall expression is very high, but again the percentage of tumor cells actually expressing $p21^{WAF1}$ significantly differs between the individual tumors. With respect to survival, both the 2- and 5-year survival rates decreased as the percentage of $p21^{WAF1}$-positive tumor cells increased. Thus defining a cut off point, patients with more than 50% positive tumor cells had a significantly worse survival rate than patients with less than 50% positive tumor cells ($p=0.0025$) (Fig. 9).

Bcl-2 Family Proteins

Among the most important regulators of apoptosis are the proteins of the Bcl-2 family. In addition to Bcl-2, which is known to be an inhibitor of programmed cell death, the family also includes Bax, Bad, Bak, Bcl-$X_{S/L}$, A1, and Mcl-1 [19], which are all proteins with either agonistic or antagonistic effects on Bcl-2. These proteins are highly conserved in four regions, the Bcl-2-homologous domains BH1–BH4, which are required for the formation of homo- and heterodimers [27]. It is accepted that cell susceptibility to apoptosis is determined by competing dimerization of the different members of the Bcl-2 family [19]. In our own immunohistochemical investigations, cytoplasmatic expression of Bax, a positive regulator of apoptosis, was demonstrated in 98.7% of all carcinomas. However, there were again striking differences concerning both the percentage of Bax-positive tumor cells and the Bax staining intensity. A score system was therefore established using these two parameters, impressively reflecting the strong heterogeneity of Bax expression between the different tumors. Bax expression was positively correlated with the grade of tumor differentiation, but there was no correlation with any of the other parameters. With respect to survival, patients with an immunoreactive score higher than the median value had a slower survival rate, but this difference did not reach statistical significance [25]. Bcl-X_L, a negative regulator of apoptosis, is also expressed in the tumor cell cytoplasm. The overall expression is very high, but using the above-mentioned score system a striking heterogeneity was also verified for Bcl-X_L expression. Similarly to Bax, Bcl-X_L was positively correlated with the grade of tumor differentiation, but there was no correlation with any of the other parameters. Concerning survival, patients with a score higher than the median value has a better survival rate than patients with a score lower than the median value ($p=0.048$) [30].

Multivariate Survival Analysis of the Molecular Candidates

In summary, out of six molecular candidates, two molecules – $p21^{WAF1}$ and Bcl-X_L – were actually correlated with patient survival. Both markers also maintained their prognostic significance in a multivariate analysis, ranking behind lymphatic vessel invasion and the new prognostic score system proposed by our group (Table 3).

Table 3. Ranking of various prognostic parameters in 149 R0 resected squamous cell carcinomas (SCC) of the esophagus

Prognostic parameter	RR	95% CI	*p* value
Lymphatic vessel invasion	1.99	1.32–3.02	0.0001
Prognostic score	1.94	1.37–2.95	0.0015
p21^{WAF1} expression	2.26	1.38–3.70	0.0032
Bcl-X_L expression	0.64	0.43–0.95	0.0119
pN category	1.55	2.04–2.33	0.0237
pT category	–	–	NS
Grading (WHO)	–	–	NS

RR, relative risk; CI, confidence interval; NS, not significant.

Molecular Parameters in Multimodally Treated Esophageal Cancer Patients

Factors influencing the result of radiochemotherapy in esophageal cancer patients have rarely been investigated so far. Furthermore, such studies have largely focused on patient- and therapy-related factors (e.g., tumor location, type of therapy) [3, 14, 20] and did not investigate the potential influence of tumor-related factors. We therefore addressed the question of whether any of the above-mentioned molecules expressed in preoperatively taken biopsies could be of value in predicting chemo- or radiosensitivity in esophageal cancer. Beginning with neoadjuvant chemotherapy, we were able to show that a high proportion of patients with p53-positive carcinomas (70.0%) did not respond to polychemotherapy, whereas in the group with p53-negative carcinomas, 45.4% did not respond. The lack of statistical significance may be due to the small number of patients investigated so far. However, the role of p53 as a predictive factor in chemosensitivity should be followed in a higher number of patients. All the other molecules investigated (p21^{WAF1}, Rb, Bcl-2, Bax, Bcl-X_L) were not predictive for chemosensitivity.

Concerning neoadjuvant radiochemotherapy, no predictive significance could be verified for any of the molecules investigated, and a promising trend could not even be detected. There was, however, a histological predictor for radiochemosensitivity: the degree of tumor differentiation according to the WHO definition. Thus we were able to show that, of the patients with poorly differentiated SCC, 87.5% responded to radiochemotherapy compared with 54.6% in the group of patients with highly or moderately differentiated carcinomas ($p=0.040$). This correlation, however, was limited to radiochemotherapy and did not apply to chemotherapy alone.

Concerning survival, we investigated the patients treated by definitive radiochemotherapy and the patients treated by radiochemotherapy and subsequent resection therapy separately (Fig. 1). Thus, in the group of patients treated by definitive radiochemotherapy, none of the molecular markers investigated correlated with survival. In contrast, in the group of patients

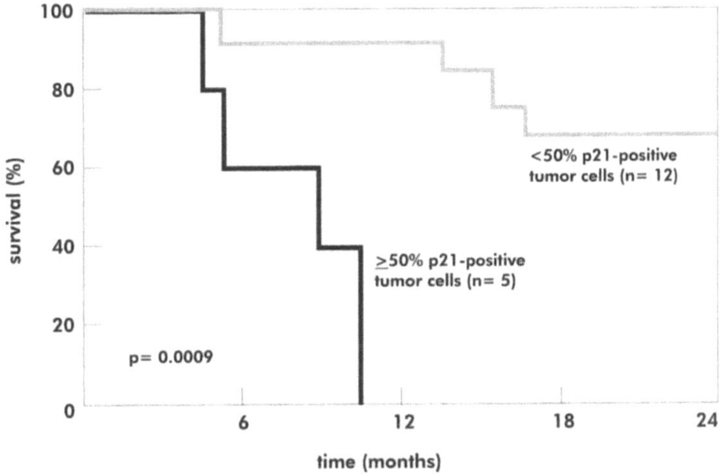

Fig. 10. Overall survival of 17 esophageal cancer patients treated by radiochemotherapy and subsequent esophageal resection in relation to $p21^{WAF1}$ expression in the tumor tissue ($p=0.0009$)

treated by radiochemotherapy and surgery, significant correlations became evident. Thus survival was significantly worse when $p21^{WAF1}$ was expressed in more than 50% of the tumor cells ($p=0.0009$) (Fig. 10), and survival was significantly worse if the tumors were positive for p53 ($p=0.0416$). No impact on survival by the other markers was observed.

Conclusions

By histological examination of surgically resected esophageal specimens parameters with strong impact on survival of esophageal cancer patients have been identified. These parameters include vascular invasion by tumor cells (blood vessel invasion and lymphatic vessel invasion), the pattern of tumor invasion and the intensity of inflammatory response at the tumor invasion front. These parameters, which provide prognostic information independent of the parameters of the TNM system are superior to the grading system as proposed by the WHO. Conventional histological examination of H&E-stained tumor sections may be extended by immunohistochemical investigations for the expression of various tumor-associated proteins. Thus, on the basis of our study the immunohistological examination for $p21^{WAF1}$ and Bcl-X_L may provide important additional prognostic information. Future clinical studies will have to show whether high risk patients as determined by the new prognostic parameters will profit from new adjuvant treatment modalities as compared with resection therapy alone.

The role of neoadjuvant treatment in the therapy of esophageal cancer has not been established yet. Although highly preliminary due to the relatively small number of patients under investigation our data suggest that immunohistochemical investigation of pretherapeutic tumor biopsies for expression of p53 and p21^{WAF1} may provide important information to the oncologist for the selection of patients for intensive combined therapy modalities with curative intention or palliative therapy.

References

1. Al-Shenebner IF, Shibata HR, Sampalis J, Jothy S (1993) Prognostic significance of proliferating cell nuclear antigen expression in colorectal cancer. Cancer 71:1954–1959
2. Cattoretti G, Becker MHG, Key G, Duchrow M, Schlüter C, Galle J, Gerdes J (1992) Monoclonal antibodies against recombinant parts of the Ki-67 antigen (MIB 1 and MIB 3) detect proliferating cells in microwave-processed formalin-fixed paraffin sections. J Pathol 168:357–363
3. Denham JW, Burmeister BH, Lamb DS, Spry NA, Joseph DJ, Hamilton CS, Yeoh E, O'Brien P, Walker QJ (1996) Factors influencing outcome following radio-chemotherapy for oesophageal cancer. Radiother Oncol 40:31–43
4. Edwards JM, Hillier VF, Lawson RAM, Mousalli H, Hasleton PS (1989) Squamous carcinoma of the oesophagus: histologic criteria and their prognostic significance. Br J Cancer 59:429–433
5. El-Deiry WS, Harper JW, O'Connor PM, Velculescu VE, Canman CE, Jackman J, Pietenpol JA, Burrel M, Hill DE, Wang Y, Wiman KG, Mercer WE, Kastan MB, Kohn KW, Elledge SJ, Kinzler KW, Vogelstein B (1994) WAF1/CIP1 is induced in p53 mediated G1 arrest and apoptosis. Cancer Res 54:1169–1174
6. Forastiere AA, Heitmiller RF, Kleinberg L (1997) Multimodality therapy for esophageal cancer. Chest 112:195S–200S
7. Gabbert HE, Meier S, Gerharz CD, Hommel G (1991) Incidence and prognostic significance of vascular invasion in 529 gastric cancer patients. Int J Cancer 49:203–207
8. Ilson DH, Kelsen DP (1994) Combined modality therapy in the treatment of esophageal cancer. Semin Oncol 21:493–507
9. International Union Against Cancer (1992) TNM classification of malignant tumours, 4th edn, 2nd rev. Springer, Berlin Heidelberg New York
10. Japanese Society for Esophageal Diseases (1976) Guidelines for the clinical and pathologic studies on carcinoma of the esophagus. Jpn J Surg 6:69–78
11. Jizuka T, Isono K, Kakegawa T, Watanabe H (1989) Parameters linked to ten-year survival in Japan of resected esophageal carcinoma. Chest 96:1005–1011
12. Kato H, Tachimori Y, Watanabe H, Jizuka T (1993) Evaluation of the new (1987) TNM classification for thoracic esophageal tumors. Int J Cancer 53:220–223
13. Kelsen DP (1997) Neoadjuvant therapy for esophageal cancer. Cancer J Sci Am 3:137–139
14. Kitamura M, Sumiyoshi K, Sonoda K, Kitamura K, Tsutsui S, Toh Y, Kuwano H, Sugimachi K (1997) The clinical and histopathological contributing factors influencing the effectiveness of preoperative hyperthermo-chemo-radiotherapy for patients with esophageal cancer. Hepatogastroenterol 44:175–180
15. Kubota Y, Petras RE, Easley KA, Bauer TW, Tubbs RR, Fazio VW (1992) Ki-67-determined growth fraction versus standard staging and grading parameters in colorectal carcinoma. Cancer 70:2602–2609
16. Lee AKC, DeLellis RA, Silverman ML, Heatly GJ, Wolfe HJ (1990) Prognostic significance of peritumoral lymphatic and blood vessel invasion in node-negative carcinoma of the breast. J Clin Oncol 8:1457–1463
17. Lowe SW (1995) Cancer therapy and p53. Curr Opin Oncol 7:547–553
18. Railo M, Nordling S, von Boguslawski K, Leivonen M, Kyllonen L, von Smitten K (1993) Prognostic value of Ki-67 immunolabelling in primary operable breast cancer. Br J Cancer 68:579–583

19. Reed JC, Miyashita T, Takayama S, Wang HG, Sato K, Krajewski S, Aime-Sempe C, Bofrug S, Kitada S, Hanada M (1996) BCL-2 family proteins: regulators of cell death involved in the pathogenesis of cancer and resistance to therapy. J Cell Biochem 60:23–32
20. Roth JA, Lichter AS, Putnam JB Jr, Forastiere AA (1993) Cancer of the esophagus. In: DeVita VT Jr, Hellmann S, Rosenberg SA (eds) Cancer: principles and practice of oncology, 4th edn. Lippincott, Philadelphia, pp 776–817
21. Sarbia M, Porschen R, Borchard F, Horstmann O, Willers R, Gabbert HE (1994) p53 protein expression and prognosis in squamous cell carcinoma of the esophagus. Cancer 74:2218–2223
22. Sarbia M, Bittinger F, Porschen R, Dutkowski P, Willers R, Gabbert HE (1995) Prognostic value of histopathologic parameters of esophageal squamous cell carcinoma. Cancer 76:922–927
23. Sarbia M, Porschen R, Borchard F, Horstmann O, Willers R, Gabbert HE (1995) Incidence and prognostic significance of vascular and neural invasion in squamous cell carcinomas of the esophagus. Int J Cancer 61:333–336
24. Sarbia M, Bittinger F, Porschen R, Dutkowski P, Torzewski M, Willers R, Gabbert HE (1996) The prognostic significance of tumour cell proliferation in squamous cell carcinomas of the oesophagus. Br J Cancer 74:1012–1016
25. Sarbia M, Bittinger F, Grabellus F, Verreet P, Dutkowski P, Willers R, Gabbert HE (1997) Expression of Bax, a proapoptotic member of the Bcl-2 family, in esophageal squamous cell carcinoma. Int J Cancer 73:508–513
26. Stahl M, Wilke H, Fink U, Stuschke M, Walz MK, Siewert JR, Molls M, Fett W, Makoski HB, Breuer N, Schmidt U, Niebel W, Sack H, Eigler FW, Seeber S (1996) Combined preoperative chemotherapy and radiotherapy in patients with locally advanced esophageal cancer; interim analysis of phase II trial. J Clin Oncol 14:829–837
27. Strasser A, Huang DCS, Vaux DL (1997) The role of the bcl-2/ced-9 gene family in cancer and general applications of defects in cell death control for tumourigenesis and resistance to chemotherapy. Biochem Biophys Acta 1333:F151–F178
28. Sugimachi K, Matsuura H, Hidenobu K, Takashi K, Kiyoshi I, Jingu K (1986) Prognostic factors of esophageal carcinoma: univariate and multivariate analyses. J Surg Oncol 31:108–112
29. Talbot IC, Ritchie S, Leighton MH, Hughes AO, Bussey HJR, Morson BC (1980) The clinical significance of invasion of veins by rectal cancer. Br J Surg 67:439–442
30. Torzewski M, Sarbia M, Heep H, Dutkowski P, Willers R, Gabbert HE (1998) Expression of Bcl-X_L an antiapoptotic member of the Bcl-2 family, in esophageal squamous cell carcinoma. Clin Cancer Res 4:577–583
31. World Health Organization (1990) Histological typing of oesophageal and gastric tumours, 2nd edn. Springer, Berlin Heidelberg New York

Malignant Progression in Barrett's Esophagus: Pathology and Molecular Biology

J. Mueller[1], M. Werner[2], J.R. Siewert[1]

[1] Chirurgische Klinik, Technische Universität München,
Klinikum rechts der Isar, Ismaninger Str. 22, 81675 Munich, Germany
[2] Pathologisches Institut, Technische Universität München,
Klinikum rechts der Isar, Ismaninger Str. 22, 81675 Munich, Germany

Abstract

Due to its increasing incidence, esophageal adenocarcinoma and its precursor lesions have received increasing attention in recent years. The histopathologic steps in the process of malignant progression in Barrett's esophagus are well described and include the following: (a) metaplasia of the normal esophageal squamous epithelium to a specialized intestinal glandular epithelium, (b) development of dysplasia (classified histologically as low and high grade), and (c) development of adenocarcinoma characterized by invasive and metastatic potential. Intestinal metaplasia can be identified by the presence of goblet cells, the detection of which can be aided by finding mucin stained by Alcian blue at low pH. Despite this well-characterized sequence, the timing of the development of dysplasia and the subsequent transition to carcinoma and the risk of development of carcinoma in low- and high-grade dysplasia are not precisely known. In addition, there are problems in the identification of dysplasia, including sampling error and interobserver discrepancies among pathologists. A better understanding of the mechanisms of these events would allow early identification and elimination of high-risk lesions before adenocarcinoma with its attendant poor prognosis were able to develop. In order to better understand this process and to potentially identify early markers of malignant transformation, a variety of molecular studies have been carried out in recent years on adenocarcinoma and its precursor lesions in Barrett's esophagus. On the phenotypic level, increased expression and changes in pattern of expression of proliferation marker (Mib-1) Ki-67 antigen, overexpression of p53 protein, overexpression of growth factors such as epidermal growth factor (EGF), c-erbB2, and transforming growth factor (TGF)-α, decreased and abnormal expression of the cell adhesion molecule E-cadherin, and, in carcinomas, increased expression of serine proteases have all been described. A new area of interest is the family of rab proteins, which play an important role in maintaining cell polarity in the gastrointestinal tract. Increased expression of one of these proteins, rab11, has been described in low-grade, but not high-grade dysplasia. In cytogenetic studies, an increased S-phase fraction, followed by an increased tetraploid (4N) fraction

Recent Results in Cancer Research, Vol. 155

and then aneuploidy, has been described. So far, the specific genes which have been most thoroughly investigated have been p53, APC, p16, and the sites of probable tumor suppressor genes, including 3p (FHIT), 13q, and 18q. With only a few exceptions (i.e., rab11 expression, and possibly mutations of FHIT), the numerous molecular abnormalities which have been described occur late in malignant progression, which means that the best marker which presently exists to identify high-risk lesions in Barrett's esophagus is the histologic identification of dysplasia in endoscopic biopsies, especially high-grade dysplasia. We are presently beginning studies using laser microdissection and competitive genomic hybridization (CGH), which could help to identify new chromosomal areas that might contain genes that are crucial in the early phases of malignant progression in Barrett's esophagus. In the future, identification of such early molecular events which predispose to carcinoma development will allow more precise and earlier risk assessment for individual patients, therefore enabling more effective therapy.

Introduction

Adenocarcinoma of the distal esophagus has the most rapidly increasing incidence among all visceral malignancies in the industrialized countries of the Western world [2, 9]. The vast majority of these tumors are thought to arise from metaplastic glandular epithelium, commonly referred to as Barrett's esophagus. Although its exact frequency in the population is uncertain, Barrett's esophagus is estimated to be found in approximately 1% of the older population and in about 3%–5% of patients with gastroesophageal reflux disease [13]. Over the past 20 years, the sequence of histomorphologic changes in the distal esophagus in response to chronic duodenogastroesophageal reflux has been well described. First, a columnar, "intestinalized" epithelium with goblet cells replaces the normal squamous epithelium of the distal esophagus in a process referred to as metaplasia [62, 63]. The presence of goblets cells is diagnostic for intestinal metaplasia and distinguishes Barrett's epithelium from normal epithelium of the proximal stomach. At times, goblet cells may be inconspicuous, and positive staining with Alcian blue at low pH (2.5) must be used to identify intestinal metaplasia. Metaplastic Barrett's epithelium is a predisposing condition for adenocarcinoma, and such patients have a 30- to 125-fold higher risk than patients without Barrett's epithelium [67]. Dysplasia in Barrett's esophagus is recognized as the precursor of adenocarcinoma and is seen morphologically as enlargement and hyperchromatism of glandular epithelial cell nuclei, increased numbers of mitoses, and loss of polarity of the cells with respect to the gland lumina along with architectural features such as crowding and increased gland complexity [21]. Depending on the severity of the changes seen, dysplasia is divided into low and high grades. Since the esophagus is easily assessable, the identification of dysplasia through a program of periodic, systematic endoscopic biopsies forms the basis for the prevention and early detection of adenocarcinoma of the esophagus [33]. Although it is known that the risk of coincident or eminent carcinoma development is high in patients with severe dysplasia [36], the timing and precise risk of carcinoma development in patients with low- and high-grade dysplasia is unclear. In addition, despite the fact that clear criteria for the identification and grading of dysplasia exist, there are problems of sampling error and interobserver differences among pathologists [54]. For this reason, when high-grade dysplasia in Barrett's esophagus is found, a pathologist with experience in this field should confirm the diagnosis [47, 55], particularly since a "prophylactic" esophagectomy is the treatment of choice in such a situation at many institutions.

The rising incidence of adenocarcinoma of the esophagus, the fact that many tumors are already advanced at the time of diagnosis, and the problems with dysplasia as a marker for the later development of carcinoma are factors which have led to intense study in order to better understand the mechanism of carcinoma development in Barrett's esophagus on the molecular level. A variety of changes along the metaplasia-dysplasia-carcinoma sequence have been described over the past several years, including gross chromosomal and DNA content errors and derangement of factors associated with cell cycle control, cell adhesion, and invasive potential. The precise timing and the impact of most of these changes are still unclear, but it is hoped that early events crucial for carcinogenesis might be identified and in the future serve as markers for early diagnosis and intervention before the carcinoma has fully developed. This review is an attempt to summarize what is presently known about the molecular events which accompany neoplastic progression in Barrett's epithelium of the esophagus.

Abnormal Protein Expression

Ki-67 Proliferation Antigen

Through immunohistochemistry a wealth of information has accumulated about the expression of proliferation marker proteins in the metaplastic, dysplastic, and carcinomatous cells of the Barrett's epithelium. In the metaplastic epithelium, Mib-1 immunohistochemistry identifies the Ki-67 proliferation antigen in the nuclei of cells within a definite proliferative zone found in the basal to midportion of the glandular epithelium. With the onset of dysplasia, this proliferative zone spreads to the surface and, in high-grade dysplasia and carcinoma, is found throughout the epithelium. Quantitative measuring of the proliferation zone as marked by Mib-1 staining has been advocated as a useful adjunct for the differentiation between low- and high-grade dysplasia [26, 49].

Growth Factors

The overexpression of a number of growth factor proteins, including fibroblast growth factor (FGF), epidermal growth factor (EGF), c-erbB2, TGF-α, and their receptors has been demonstrated in adenocarcinoma of the distal esophagus. In particular, acidic FGF has been reported to accumulate along the sequence from low- to high-grade dysplasia and carcinoma [61] and could be useful as one of a panel of markers for the identification of high-grade dysplasia in biopsies. A total of 64% of esophageal adenocarcinomas are reported to express EGF receptor (EGFR), and this factor has been correlated with poor patient survival [69].

Fas/APO-1 (CD95)

Apoptosis and its control has gained increasing recognition as an important factor in the loss of tumor proliferation control in carcinogenesis. Fas/APO-1 (CD95) is a membrane-associated protein which serves as the receptor for Fas-ligand. Binding of Fas-ligand with its receptor elicits a signal which results in apoptosis. The loss of Fas expression has been shown to be a common mechanism in a variety of tumors, causing an interruption in the apoptotic pathway [43]. Recently, an abnormality in Fas expression was observed in adenocarcinomas arising in Barrett's epithelium in which the immunohistochemical staining for Fas at the cell surface was reduced or absent despite a high level of Fas mRNA detected by Northern blotting [27]. In addition, an esophageal adenocarcinoma cell line showed an abnormal accumulation of Fas protein in the cell cytoplasm along with a lack of localization on the cell surface. In this way, the tumor cells may be able to avoid the normal controls which maintain the balance between cell proliferation and death.

Adhesion Molecules: E-Cadherin and the Catenins

Adhesion molecules are known to play crucial roles in the attachment of epithelial cells to one another and to their extracellular matrix. The processes of invasion and metastasis, which are central to the development of the malignant phenotype, are closely associated with reduction or loss of cell adhesion protein expression [8]. E-cadherin is a transmembrane molecule which mediates cell-cell adhesion and is dependent on a cytoplasmic interaction with α-, β-, and γ-catenin for its connection to the actin cytoskeleton. In one recent study, a statistically significant reduction of E-cadherin and of α- and β-catenin protein expression was found by immunohistochemistry in both low- and high-grade dysplasia, as well as in carcinoma [66]. This indicates that the disruption of the normal cell-cell contact is an important process in early carcinogenesis in Barrett's epithelium. In a second study, which concentrated on adenocarcinoma arising in Barrett's epithelium, 70% of patients showed a strong reduction in both E-cadherin and catenin, which suggests that the expression of these molecules is closely related [31]. This study also found that the reduction in both E-cadherin and beta catenin were significantly related to poor survival, regardless of tumor stage. Either gene mutation or abnormalities of the transcription and translation of the cadherin and catenin genes may account for this abnormal expression [7, 11]. Alternatively, disturbances of the normal interaction between cadherin and catenin proteins and other molecules which are commonly involved in carcinogenesis (EGFR, c-erbB2, or APC) may be the source of these abnormalities [1].

Cell Polarity: rab11

Related to the intercellular organization of epithelia mediated by adhesion molecules is the intracellular organization of cell organelles and vesicles with respect to the basal and apical cell membranes, an important aspect of cell polarity. Mediators of cell polarity include the rab family, a class of GTP-binding proteins which were first described in 1993 [19] and have been found to be distributed throughout the gastrointestinal tract. Interestingly, abnormalities of the expression of rab11, a member of this family, have been recently found in Barrett's epithelium. Ray et al. [51] described that the metaplastic, intestinalized epithelia of Barrett's esophagus shows only faint, perinuclear immunostaining for Rab11, whereas strong staining is seen in the supranuclear area in cells in areas of low-grade dysplasia. In both highly dysplastic and carcinomatous cells, staining is again very weak or absent. This finding may be an insight into the molecular basis for the development of the dysplastic phenotype in Barrett's esophagus and, in a panel of antibodies, could serve as a useful marker to differentiate between low- and high-grade dysplasia.

Proteases

During the process of invasion and metastasis, tumor cells must be able to degrade their surrounding extracellular matrix. Important mediators of this degradation include the serine protease family, which has been extensively studied in a variety of tumor types as potential prognostic markers [56]. The serine proteases are apparently expressed in detectable amounts only once invasion is histologically evident, but so far, no systematic study of their expression in metaplastic or dysplastic Barrett's epithelium has been published. For esophageal adenocarcinomas which have been completely resected, high levels of urokinase-like plasminogen activator (UPA), as detected by enzyme-linked immunosorbent analysis (ELISA) performed on tumor tissue samples, was found to be an independent prognostic indicator of subsequent poor survival [44].

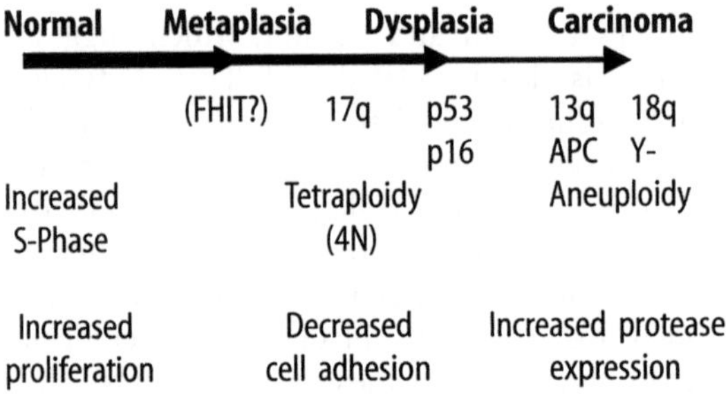

Fig. 1. A summary of the histopathologic and molecular changes accompanying malignant progression in Barrett's esophagus

Abnormal DNA Content

In Barrett's epithelium, a sequence of DNA content changes has been identified along the metaplasia-dysplasia-carcinoma sequence beginning with an increased S-phase in metaplasia, an increased tetraploid (4N) fraction and then, in patients with high-grade dysplasia and carcinoma, aneuploidy [53] (Fig. 1). Aneuploidy, or abnormal DNA content, is a finding which accompanies tumor development and progression in a wide variety of tumor types. The majority of Barrett's adenocarcinomas have been found to be aneuploid [16], and since aneuploidy can be detected with an automated, flow cytometric system, its detection has been proposed as screening method in support of histopathology for identifying patients at high risk for having or developing malignancy [34]. Flow cytometry has also identified multiple aneuploid clones in dysplastic Barrett's epithelium, suggesting that the genome of the metaplastic mucosa of these patients is unstable [50]. Some problems with the detection of aneuploidy have been described in the literature, including false-positive results caused by delayed processing of fresh tissue specimens [40] and a lack of detection by flow cytometry in histopathologic biopsies showing dysplasia [58], which might have been due to sampling problems or to the fact that a minority of adenocarcinomas of the esophagus are diploid.

Cytogenetics

Cytogenetic studies of adenocarcinomas arising in Barrett's esophagus have revealed frequent losses of chromosomes 4, 18, 21, and Y, and frequent gains of chromosomes 14 and 20. Chromosomal arms 1p, 3p, 3q, 11p, and 22p have the most frequent structural abnormalities [37]. Descriptions of the cytogenetics of dysplastic and metaplastic Barrett's epithelium using classical cytogenetic techniques do not exist, due to the problems with precise epithelial tissue sampling.

Specific Genetic Abnormalities

Newer molecular techniques have allowed precise identification of genes and chromosomal areas which play, or could potentially play, important roles in tumor development and progression in Barrett's esophagus. The most notable are briefly reviewed.

p53

p53 is the most extensively studied gene with respect to tumor development and progression in nearly every tumor type, and adenocarcinoma arising in Barrett's esophagus is no exception. Located on chromosome 17p, the p53 gene is transcribed in response to DNA damage. Wild-type p53 protein delays the cell cycle long enough so that DNA repair can take place. If the DNA damage cannot be repaired, p53 drives the cell into apoptosis. The inactivation and loss of function of p53 is a key event in carcinogenesis which promotes genetic instability and further uncontrolled damage and cell proliferation. According to the "two hit" theory of Knudson, two events (mutation of one allele and deletion of the second) are needed to inactivate p53 [24, 32]. Immunohistochemical detection of p53 is based on the fact that the mutated molecule often accumulates in the nucleus. However, since non-mutated p53 may also accumulate enough to become detectable by sensitive immunohistochemical methods and some mutations result in loss of p53 transcription, more precise methods such as single-strand conformation polymorphism (SSCP) followed by sequencing are needed to definitely identify p53 mutations [28].

In contrast to the numerous studies of p53 in adenocarcinoma arising in Barrett's esophagus, there are few studies which have applied mutational analysis of p53 to areas of metaplasia and dysplasia. p53 mutations have occasionally been reported to be detectable in metaplasia or low-grade dysplasia, indicating that mutation of p53 is an early event [12]. In both high-grade dysplasia and adenocarcinoma, the frequency of p53 mutation has been found in several studies to be approximately 60% [3, 18, 23, 28, 45, 57]. It has been hypothesized that p53 mutation is an event in the progression to carcinoma in Barrett's esophagus which follows an increased S-phase and tetraploid (4N) fraction, but precedes and is the initiator of aneuploidy, and thereby functions as the switch in the transition from low- to high-grade dysplasia [52]. Some 69% of p53 mutations in Barrett's adenocarcinomas have been found to be CpG transitions [25], far higher than any other tumor type studied thus far [39]. The cause and biologic significance of this unique finding are unknown.

The majority of studies of p53 in Barrett's esophagus are descriptions of immunohistochemical results using paraffin sections. In general, the results are comparable to the studies using mutational analysis, but usually show a higher prevalence of p53 protein accumulation than would be expected from the mutation rate. An increased rate of p53 staining is seen along the pathway from metaplasia to dysplasia to carcinoma, and immunohistochemistry for p53 has therefore been proposed as a marker of progression in Barrett's esophagus [29, 30]. Used together with other antibodies, p53 could be helpful for the distinction between low- and high-grade dysplasia [49]. There have been some reports that positive immunohistochemistry for p53 might be an indicator of poor prognosis for patients with adenocarcinoma of the esophagus [42], but so far these data are inconclusive.

APC

The APC (adenomatous polyposis coli) gene on chromosome 5q is a key tumor suppressor gene in the early stages of carcinogenesis in the colorectum [15], in particular since it plays a key role in the development of colonic adenomas [60]. In Barrett's esophagus, the situation appears to be different, since most studies show that APC abnormalities are late in the progression to invasive cancer, being either coincident with [20], or subsequent to p53 mutation [10]. Although loss of heterozygosity (LOH) at 5q is frequently found in esophageal adenocarcinoma, the results for metaplasia and dysplasia are conflicting. One study failed to detect any LOH at 5q in dysplastic tissue [20], but contamination by normal tissue may have been a problem since microdissection was not used. A second study by Zhuang et al. [70] showed allelic loss at the APC locus in both metaplastic and dysplastic areas in close proximity to carcinoma, suggesting that this LOH identified a clone which later progressed to carcinoma.

p16

The p16 (CDKN2A, INK44A, or MTS1) protein inhibits cell proliferation by preventing cyclin-dependent kinases from inactivating the Rb (retinoblastoma) gene product by phosphorylation [59]. Inactivation of the p16 gene on 9p21 by mutation, deletion, or hypermethylation allows uncontrolled cell proliferation [35]. p16 gene inactivation is described in the progression to Barrett's adenocarcinoma, but seems to be a late event [20, 68]. In one study, however, allelic loss at 9p21 seemed to precede the development of aneuploidy in areas of dysplasia in Barrett's epithelium [5], suggesting a role for p16 abnormalities in the promotion of genetic instability, similar to p53.

Other Tumor Suppressor Genes

The microsatellite analysis method, which utilizes polymorphic markers at multiple loci, is an excellent means of identifying allelic loss, usually referred to as LOH. When a consistent LOH is seen in a tumor entity at a specific chromosomal location, the presence of a tumor suppressor gene at that site can be suspected. In studies of adenocarcinomas arising in Barrett's esophagus, the highest rates of LOH are found on chromosome arms 3p, 4q, 5q, 6q, 9p, 12q, 17p, 17q, and 18q [4, 17, 65]. Some of these sites are the locations of known genes, e.g., 5q – APC, 9p – p16, and 17p – p53, but others may contain genes which are not yet identified or identified genes which are not yet known to play a role in carcinogenesis in Barrett's esophagus.

One area of particular interest is the 18q chromosomal arm. Loss of the 18q21.1 region has been found in 45% of samples of aneuploid Barrett's adenocarcinoma and in 46% of samples of aneuploid dysplastic epithelium [6]. Since this LOH was also found in three quarters of diploid tissue samples, it appears that this may be an early event which precedes the development of aneuploidy and carcinoma. Two possible target genes in this are the DPC4 gene (deleted in pancreatic carcinoma, locus 4), which is inactivated by homozygous deletion in approximately 30% of pancreatic adenocarcinomas [6, 22], and DCC (deleted in colorectal cancer) [4, 6].

Another region of interest in Barrett's adenocarcinoma showing frequent allelic loss is 3p14.2. This is of interest since FHIT (fragile histidine triad gene), a presumptive tumor suppressor gene is found at this site [46]. The function of the FHIT protein is not known, but the FHIT gene spans the fragile site FRA3B and is thus predisposed to develop structural chromosomal aberrations such as translocations or deletions, especially following exposure to toxins [64]. The reverse transcriptase-polymerase chain reaction (RT-PCR) has detected exon deletion of FHIT mRNA in up to 86% of metaplasia and in 93% of adenocarcinomas [14, 38, 71], which would indicate that this is a very early event in carcinogenesis in Barrett's epithelium. However, homozygous deletions of the genomic DNA have been found only in invasive cancer and involve large regions [38], and different patterns of transcript aberration have been seen in paired non-neoplastic and neoplastic samples [14], findings which indicate that FHIT may not be the target suppressor gene in this area. Exposure to toxins may lead to widespread genomic damage on the 3p arm due to the fragile site, and any of a number of, as yet, unidentified suppressor genes at this site could be more important in tumor progression in Barrett's esophagus [14].

Recently, a putative tumor suppressor gene found on the distal portion of the 17q chromosomal arm was identified which appears to be important in the development of squamous cell carcinoma of the esophagus [41]. An investigation of adenocarcinomas arising in Barrett's epithelium showed an LOH of this region in both carcinoma and matched metaplasia samples in over half of the informative cases [48], suggesting that this region may also be an early event in esophageal adenocarcinoma development.

Future Directions

There has been considerable progress in our understanding of the molecular biology of neoplastic progression in Barrett's esophagus. A variety of changes at the DNA, RNA, and protein levels have been described which accompany the metaplasia-dysplasia-carcinoma sequence. Although a few of these changes appear quite early along this pathway (e.g., increased S-phase fraction, increased rab11 expression), the majority are late and are only found once high-grade dysplasia or even carcinoma are already evident. This means that, at present, combinations of these markers and changes can be helpful for clinicopathologic decision-making, but that a systematic endoscopic biopsy program with the identification of dysplasia remains the gold standard to identify patients at high risk for adenocarcinoma development. In the future, identification of the early, crucial molecular events in neoplastic progression will lead not only to a more accurate, earlier risk assessment for the individual patient, but may also provide us with targets for specific intervention to prevent the development of dysplasia and carcinoma.

References

1. al-Kasspooles M, Moore JH, Orringer MB, Beer DG (1993) Amplification and over-expression of the EGFR and erbB-2 genes in human esophageal adenocarcinomas. Int J Cancer 54:213–219
2. Altorki NK, Oliveria S, Schrump DS (1997) Epidemiology and molecular biology of Barrett's adenocarcinoma. Semin Surg Oncol 13:270–280
3. Audrezet MP, Robaszkiewicz M, Mercier B, Nousbaum JB, Hardy E, Bail JP, Volant A, Lozac'h P, Gouerou H, Ferec C (1996) Molecular analysis of the TP53 gene in Barrett's adenocarcinoma. Hum Mutat 7:109–113
4. Barrett MT, Galipeau PC, Sanchez CA, Emond MJ, Reid BJ (1996) Determination of the frequency of loss of heterozygosity in esophageal adenocarcinoma by cell sorting, whole genome amplification and microsatellite polymorphisms. Oncogene 12:1873–1878
5. Barrett MT, Sanchez CA, Galipeau PC, Neshat K, Emond M, Reid BJ (1996) Allelic loss of 9p21 and mutation of the CDKN2/p16 gene develop as early lesions during neoplastic progression in Barrett's esophagus. Oncogene 13:1867–1873
6. Barrett MT, Schutte M, Kern SE, Reid BJ (1996) Allelic loss and mutational analysis of the DPC4 gene in esophageal adenocarcinoma. Cancer Res 56:4351–4353
7. Becker KF, Atkinson MJ, Reich U, Becker I, Nekarda H, Siewert JR, Hofler H (1994) E-cadherin gene mutations provide clues to diffuse type gastric carcinomas. Cancer Res 54:3845–3852
8. Behrens J (1994) Cadherins as determinants of tissue morphology and suppressors of invasion. Acta Anat (Basel) 149:165–169
9. Blot WJ, Devesa SS, Kneller RW, Fraumeni JF Jr (1991) Rising incidence of adenocarcinoma of the esophagus and gastric cardia. JAMA 265:1287–1289
10. Blount PL, Meltzer SJ, Yin J, Huang Y, Krasna MJ, Reid BJ (1993) Clonal ordering of 17p and 5q allelic losses in Barrett dysplasia and adenocarcinoma. Proc Natl Acad Sci USA 90:3221–3225
11. Breen E, Clarke A, Steele G Jr, Mercurio AM (1993) Poorly differentiated colon carcinoma cell lines deficient in alpha-catenin expression express high levels of surface E-cadherin but lack Ca(2+)-dependent cell-cell adhesion. Cell Adhes Commun 1:239–250
12. Casson AG, Manolopoulos B, Troster M, Kerkvliet N, O'Malley F, Inculet R, Finley R, Roth JA (1994) Clinical implications of p53 gene mutation in the progression of Barrett's epithelium to invasive esophageal cancer. Am J Surg 167:52–57
13. Chen MY, Ott DJ, Gelfand DW (1995) More evidence for the increasing prevalence of adenocarcinoma of the esophagus over an 18-year period. J Clin Gastroenterol 21:254–255

14. Chen YJ, Chen PH, Lee MD, Chang JG (1997) Aberrant FHIT transcripts in cancerous and corresponding non-cancerous lesions of the digestive tract. Int J Cancer 72:955–958
15. Fearon ER, Vogelstein B (1990) A genetic model for colorectal tumorigenesis. Cell 61:759–767
16. Giaretti W (1997) Aneuploidy mechanisms in human colorectal preneoplastic lesions and Barrett's esophagus. Is there a role for K-ras and p53 mutations? Anal Cell Pathol 15:99–117
17. Gleeson CM, Sloan JM, McGuigan JA (1995) Multiple gene alterations in esophageal adenocarcinoma. Proc Ann Meet Am Assoc Cancer Res 6:3251A
18. Gleeson CM, Sloan JM, McGuigan JA, Ritchie AJ, Russell SE (1995) Base transitions at CpG dinucleotides in the p53 gene are common in esophageal adenocarcinoma. Cancer Res 55:3406–3411
19. Goldenring JR, Shen KR, Vaughan HD, Modlin IM (1993) Identification of a small GTP-binding protein, Rab25, expressed in the gastrointestinal mucosa, kidney, and lung. J Biol Chem 268:18419–18422
20. Gonzalez MV, Artimez ML, Rodrigo L, Lopez-Larrea C, Menendez MJ, Alvarez V, Perez R, Fresno MF, Perez MJ, Sampedro A, Coto E (1997) Mutation analysis of the p53, APC, and p16 genes in the Barrett's oesophagus, dysplasia, and adenocarcinoma. J Clin Pathol 50:212–217
21. Haggitt RC (1994) Barrett's esophagus, dysplasia, and adenocarcinoma. Hum Pathol 25:982–993
22. Hahn SA, Schutte M, Hoque AT, Moskaluk CA, da Costa LT, Rozenblum E, Weinstein CL, Fischer A, Yeo CJ, Hruban RH, Kern SE (1996) DPC4, a candidate tumor suppressor gene at human chromosome 18q21.1. Science 271:350–353
23. Hamelin R, Flejou JF, Muzeau F, Potet F, Laurent-Puig P, Fekete F, Thomas G (1994) TP53 gene mutations and p53 protein immunoreactivity in malignant and premalignant Barrett's esophagus. Gastroenterology 107:1012–1018
24. Hartwell L (1992) Defects in a cell cycle checkpoint may be responsible for the genomic instability of cancer cells. Cell 71:543–546
25. Hollstein M, Shomer B, Greenblatt M, Soussi T, Hovig E, Montesano R, Harris CC (1996) Somatic point mutations in the p53 gene of human tumors and cell lines: updated compilation. Nucleic Acids Res 24:141–146
26. Hong MK, Laskin WB, Herman BE, Johnston MH, Vargo JJ, Steinberg SM, Allegra CJ, Johnston PG (1995) Expansion of the Ki-67 proliferative compartment correlates with degree of dysplasia in Barrett's esophagus. Cancer 75:423–429
27. Hughes SJ, Nambu Y, Soldes OS, Hamstra D, Rehemtulla A, Iannettoni MD, Orringer MB, Beer DG (1997) Fas/APO-1 (CD95) is not translocated to the cell membrane in esophageal adenocarcinoma. Cancer Res 57:5571–5578
28. Ireland AP, Clark GW, DeMeester TR (1997) Barrett's esophagus. The significance of p53 in clinical practice. Ann Surg 225:17–30
29. Jones DR, Davidson AG, Summers CL, Murray GF, Quinlan DC (1994) Potential application of p53 as an intermediate biomarker in Barrett's esophagus. Ann Thorac Surg 57:598–603
30. Krishnadath KK, Tilanus HW, van Blankenstein M, Bosman FT, Mulder AH (1995) Accumulation of p53 protein in normal, dysplastic, and neoplastic Barrett's oesophagus. J Pathol 175:175–180
31. Krishnadath KK, Tilanus HW, van Blankenstein M, Hop WC, Kremers ED, Dinjens WN, Bosman FT (1997) Reduced expression of the cadherin-catenin complex in oesophageal adenocarcinoma correlates with poor prognosis. J Pathol 182:331–338
32. Levine AJ (1992) The p53 tumor-suppressor gene. N Engl J Med 326:1350–1352
33. Levine DS, Haggitt RC, Blount PL, Rabinovitch PS, Rusch VW, Reid BJ (1993) An endoscopic biopsy protocol can differentiate high-grade dysplasia from early adenocarcinoma in Barrett's esophagus. Gastroenterology 105:40–50
34. Lewin KJ, Appelman HD (1996) Tumors of the esophagus and stomach. Atlas of tumor pathology, 3rd series, 3rd edn. Armed Forces Institute of Pathology, Washington DC

35. Lukas J, Parry D, Aagaard L, Mann DJ, Bartkova J, Strauss M, Peters G, Bartek J (1995) Retinoblastoma-protein-dependent cell-cycle inhibition by the tumour suppressor p16. Nature 375:503–506
36. McArdle JE, Lewin KJ, Randall G, Weinstein W (1992) Distribution of dysplasias and early invasive carcinoma in Barrett's esophagus. Hum Pathol 23:479–482
37. Menke-Pluymers MB, van Drunen E, Vissers KJ, Mulder AH, Tilanus HW, Hagemeijer A (1996) Cytogenetic analysis of Barrett's mucosa and adenocarcinoma of the distal esophagus and cardia. Cancer Genet Cytogenet 90:109–117
38. Michael D, Beer DG, Wilke CW, Miller DE, Glover TW (1997) Frequent deletions of FHIT and FRA3B in Barrett's metaplasia and esophageal adenocarcinomas. Oncogene 15:1653–1659
39. Montesano R, Hollstein M, Hainaut P (1996) Genetic alterations in esophageal cancer and their relevance to etiology and pathogenesis: a review. Int J Cancer 69:225–235
40. Montgomery EA, Hartmann DP, Carr NJ, Holterman DA, Sobin LH, Azumi N (1996) Barrett esophagus with dysplasia. Flow cytometric DNA analysis of routine, paraffin-embedded mucosal biopsies. Am J Clin Pathol 106:298–304
41. Mori T, Aoki T, Matsubara T, Iida F, Du X, Nishihira T, Mori S, Nakamura Y (1994) Frequent loss of heterozygosity in the region including BRCA1 on chromosome 17q in squamous cell carcinomas of the esophagus. Cancer Res 54:1638–1640
42. Moskaluk CA, Heitmiller R, Zahurak M, Schwab D, Sidransky D, Hamilton SR (1996) p53 and p21(WAF1/CIP1/SDI1) gene products in Barrett esophagus and adenocarcinoma of the esophagus and esophagogastric junction. Hum Pathol 27:1211–1220
43. Nagata S, Goldstein P (1995) The Fas death factor. Science 267:1449–1456
44. Nekarda H, Schmitt M, Schlegel P, Stark M, Becker K, Mueller J, Siewert JR (1998) Strong prognostic impact of tumor-associated urokinase-type plasminogen activator (uPA) in completely resected adenocarcinoma of the esophagus. Clin Cancer Res 4:1755–1763
45. Neshat K, Sanchez CA, Galipeau PC, Blount PL, Levine DS, Joslyn G, Reid BJ (1994) p53 mutations in Barrett's adenocarcinoma and high-grade dysplasia. Gastroenterology 106:1589–1595
46. Ohta M, Inoue H, Cotticelli MG, Kastury K, Baffa R, Palazzo J, Siprashvili Z, Mori M, McCue P, Druck T (1996) The FHIT gene, spanning the chromosome 3p14.2 fragile site and renal carcinoma-associated t(3;8) breakpoint, is abnormal in digestive tract cancers. Cell 84:587–597
47. Pera M, Trastek VF, Carpenter HA, Allen MS, Deschamps C, Pairolero PC (1992) Barrett's esophagus with high-grade dysplasia: an indication for esophagectomy? Ann Thorac Surg 54:199–204
48. Petty EM, Kalikin LM, Orringer MB, Beer DG (1998) Distal chromosome 17q loss in Barrett's esophageal and gastric cardia adenocarcinomas: implications for tumorigenesis. Mol Carcinog 22:222–228
49. Polkowski W, Baak JPA, Van Lanshot JJB, Meijer GA, Schuurmans LT, Ten Kate FJW, Obertrop H, Offerhaus GJA (1998) Clinical decision making in Barrett's oesophagus can be supported by computerized immunoquantitation and morphometry of features associated with proliferation and differentiation. J Pathol 184:161–168
50. Rabinovitch PS, Reid BJ, Haggitt RC, Norwood TH, Rubin CE (1989) Progression to cancer in Barrett's esophagus is associated with genomic instability. Lab Invest 60:65–71
51. Ray GS, Lee JR, Nwokeji K, Mills LR, Goldenring JR (1997) Increased immunoreactivity for Rab11, a small GTP-binding protein, in low-grade dysplastic Barrett's epithelia. Lab Invest 77:503–511
52. Reid BJ, Barrett MT, Galipeau PC, Sanchez CA, Neshat K, Cowan DS, Levine DS (1996) Barrett's esophagus: ordering the events that lead to cancer. Eur J Cancer Prev 5 [Suppl 2]:57–65
53. Reid BJ, Blount PL, Rubin CE, Levine DS, Haggitt RC, Rabinovitch PS (1992) Flow-cytometric and histological progression to malignancy in Barrett's esophagus: prospective endoscopic surveillance of a cohort. Gastroenterology 102:1212–1219

54. Reid BJ, Haggitt RC, Rubin CE, Roth G, Surawicz CM, Van Belle G, Lewin K, Weinstein WM, Antonioli DA, Goldman H (1988) Observer variation in the diagnosis of dysplasia in Barrett's esophagus. Hum Pathol 19:166–178
55. Rusch VW, Levine DS, Haggitt R, Reid BJ (1994) The management of high grade dysplasia and early cancer in Barrett's esophagus. A multidisciplinary problem. Cancer 74:1225–1229
56. Schmitt M, Wilhelm O, Janicke F, Magdolen V, Reuning U, Ohi H, Moniwa N, Kobayashi H, Weidle U, Graeff H (1995) Urokinase-type plasminogen activator (uPA) and its receptor (CD87): a new target in tumor invasion and metastasis. J Obstet Gynaecol 21:151–165
57. Schneider PM, Casson AG, Levin B, Garewal HS, Hoelscher AH, Becker K, Dittler HJ, Cleary KR, Troster M, Siewert JR, Roth JA (1996) Mutations of p53 in Barrett's esophagus and Barrett's cancer: a prospective study of ninety-eight cases. J Thorac Cardiovasc Surg 111:323–331
58. Sciallero S, Giaretti W, Bonelli L, Geido E, Rapallo A, Conio M, Ravelli P, Lombardo L, Briglia R, Lapertosa G (1993) DNA content analysis of Barrett's esophagus by flow cytometry. Endoscopy 25:648–651
59. Serrano M, Hannon GJ, Beach D (1993) A new regulatory motif in cell-cycle control causing specific inhibition of cyclin D/CDK4. Nature 366:704–707
60. Shibata H, Toyama K, Shioya H, Ito M, Hirota M, Hasegawa S, Matsumoto H, Takano H, Akiyama T, Toyoshima K, Kanamaru R, Kanegae Y, Saito I, Nakamura Y, Shiba K, Noda T (1997) Rapid colorectal adenoma formation initiated by conditional targeting of the Apc gene. Science 278:120–123
61. Soslow RA, Ying L, Altorki NK (1997) Expression of acidic fibroblast growth factor in Barrett's esophagus and associated esophageal adenocarcinoma. J Thorac Cardiovasc Surg 114:838–843
62. Spechler SJ, Goyal RK (1986) Barrett's esophagus. N Engl J Med 315:362–371
63. Stein HJ, Panel of experts (1998) Epidemiology, classification, pathogenesis, pathology, and surveillance for adenocarcinoma of the esophagogastric junction. Results of a Consensus Conference of the International Society for Diseases of the Esophagus and International Gastric Cancer Association. Dis Esophagus (in press)
64. Sutherland GR (1991) Chromosomal fragile sites. Genet Anal Tech Appl 8:161–166
65. Swift A, Risk JM, Kingsnorth AN, Wright TA, Myskow M, Field JK (1995) Frequent loss of heterozygosity on chromosome 17 at 17q11.2-q12 in Barrett's adenocarcinoma. Br J Cancer 71:995–998
66. Washington K, Chiappori A, Hamilton K, Shyr Y, Blanke C, Johnson D, Sawyers J, Beauchamp D (1998) Expression of beta-catenin, alpha-catenin, and E-cadherin in Barrett's esophagus and esophageal adenocarcinomas. Mod Pathol 11:805–813
67. Williamson WA, Ellis FH Jr, Gibb SP, Shahian DM, Aretz HT, Heatley GJ, Watkins E Jr (1991) Barrett's esophagus. Prevalence and incidence of adenocarcinoma. Arch Intern Med 151:2212–2216
68. Wong DJ, Barrett MT, Stoger R, Emond MJ, Reid BJ (1997) p16INK4a promoter is hypermethylated at a high frequency in esophageal adenocarcinomas. Cancer Res 57:2619–2622
69. Yacoub L, Goldman H, Odze RD (1997) Transforming growth factor-alpha, epidermal growth factor receptor, and MiB-1 expression in Barrett's-associated neoplasia: correlation with prognosis. Mod Pathol 10:105–112
70. Zhuang Z, Vortmeyer AO, Mark EJ, Odze R, Emmert-Buck MR, Merino MJ, Moon H, Liotta LA, Duray PH (1996) Barrett's esophagus: metaplastic cells with loss of heterozygosity at the APC gene locus are clonal precursors to invasive adenocarcinoma. Cancer Res 56:1961–1964
71. Zou TT, Lei J, Shi YQ, Yin J, Wang S, Souza RF, Kong D, Shimada Y, Smolinski KN, Greenwald BD, Abraham JM, Harpaz N, Meltzer SJ (1997) FHIT gene alterations in esophageal cancer and ulcerative colitis (UC). Oncogene 15:101–105

Malignant Degeneration of Barrett's Esophagus: Clinical Point of View

H.J. Stein, M. Feith, J.R. Siewert

Chirurgische Klinik und Poliklinik, Klinikum rechts der Isar der TU München, Ismaningerstr. 22, 81675 Munich, Germany

Abstract

The incidence of adenocarcinoma of the distal esophagus is increasing at an alarming rate. Intestinal metaplasia in the distal esophagus, i.e. Barrett's esophagus, has been identified as the single most important risk factor for these tumors. Barrett's esophagus develops as a consequence of chronic mucosal injury in up to 10% of patients with long-lasting gastroesophageal reflux disease. Experimental and clinical data indicate that adenocarcinoma of the distal esophagus is a direct consequence of mixed (i.e., acid and bile) reflux into the esophagus. Interestingly, *Helicobacter pylori* infection of the stomach appears to exert a protective effect against the development of esophageal adenocarcinoma. Neither aggressive medical acid suppression nor antireflux surgery can induce a predictable regression of Barrett's esophagus or exert a protective effect against its malignant degeneration. Endoscopic ablation of Barrett's esophagus, although appealing, currently constitutes a potentially dangerous procedure without proven benefit for the patient. Since the development of Barrett's adenocarcinoma follows a multistep process from metaplasia through increasingly severe grades of dysplasia, close endoscopic surveillance with extensive biopsies currently remains the only means to identify patients at risk for malignant degeneration and detect esophageal adenocarcinoma at an early and curable stage.

Introduction

Esophageal adenocarcinoma was an uncommon entity before 1970. Since then the incidence and prevalence of adenocarcinoma of the esophagus has risen dramatically in North America and Western Europe [1, 2, 10]. Population based studies in the U.S. and several European countries indicate that the incidence of esophageal adenocarcinoma has doubled between the early 1970s and the late 1980s and continues to increase at a rate of about 5% to 10% per year [10]. This is paralleled by rising rates of adenocarcinoma of the gastric cardia and subcardial gastric carcinoma. Blot et al. have stated

Recent Results in Cancer Research, Vol. 155

that the rate of increase of esophageal and esophago-gastric junction adenocarcinoma in the U.S. during the past decade surpassed that of any other type of cancer [1]. In the mid 1990s the incidence of oesophageal adenocarcinoma has been estimated between 1 and 4 per 100000 and year in the U.S. and several European countries and has thus surpassed that of squamous cell esophageal cancer in these countries. In Asia and Africa adenocarcinoma of the esophagus still constitutes an uncommon finding. However, reports on increasing rates for esophago-gastric junction adenocarcinoma are also emerging from these areas.

Most, if not all adenocarcinomas of the distal esophagus arise from areas with intestinal metaplasia, i.e. the so-called Barrett's esophagus. Several prospective studies have shown that the estimated risk for the development of an esophageal adenocarcinoma in patients with known Barrett's esophagus of more than 3 cm in length is increased about 100-fold as compared to the general population [31, 34]. In these patients the annual risk for developing an esophageal adenocarcinoma has been estimated to be about 1%. This translates into a life-time esophageal adenocarcinoma risk of about 10% in patients with Barrett's esophagus of more than 3 cm in length [31]. Barrett's esophagus has thus been identified as the single most important precursor lesion for adenocarcinoma of the distal esophagus.

More recently, adenocarcinoma of the gastric cardia and subcardial gastric cancer have also been linked to the presence of short segments with intestinal metaplasia in the distal esophagus or at the esophago-gastric junction [7]. It currently remains, unclear whether intestinal metaplasia at the esophago-gastric junction without macroscopic evidence for columnar cell lining of the esophagus, and short or long segments with intestinal metaplasia in the distal esophagus represent a continuum of the same underlying disease process or constitute different entities [30, 32]. This is largely due to the ambiguous use of the term "Barrett's esophagus" in many studies without a description and differentiation of the assessed conditions. A clear differentiation of patients with foci of intestinal metaplasia at or below the esophago-gastric junction but no endoscopic evidence of columnar cell lining of the distal esophagus, patients with segments or tongues of intestinal metaplasia in the distal esophagus shorter than 3 cm in length (the so-called short segment Barrett's esophagus), and patients with greater than 3 cm segments of specialized intestinal metaplasia in the distal esophagus (the so-called long segment or classic Barrett's esophagus) appears reasonable in future studies [20, 31, 32].

Malignant Degeneration of Barrett's Esophagus: Clinical Issues

Gastroesophageal Reflux, Barrett's Esophagus and Barrett's Cancer

Intestinal metaplasia of the esophagus, i.e., Barrett's esophagus, develops when the normal squamous esophageal epithelium is replaced by columnar epithelium during the process of healing after acute injury to the squamous esophageal mucosa [31, 33]. In most patients with Barrett's esophagus, chronic gastroesophageal reflux is the underlying abnormality causing acute mucosal injury and providing the abnormal environment during the healing process which predisposes to intestinal metaplasia [33, 34]. A recent nationwide, population-based, case-control study in Sweden showed an odds ratio of 7.7 for esophageal adenocarcinoma in persons with recurrent reflux symptoms, as compared with persons without such symptoms [15]. The more frequent, more severe, and longer-lasting the symptoms of reflux, the greater the risk. Among persons with long-standing and severe symptoms of reflux, the odds ratio for esophageal adenocarcinoma was 43.5. Based on these data, there is a strong and probably causal relation between gastroesophageal reflux, one of the most common benign disorders of the digestive tract, and esophageal adenocarcinoma. However, only about 10% of patients with gastroesophageal reflux disease develop intestinal metaplasia and only about 10% of these patients progress to esophageal adenocarcinoma. Early identification of the subgroup of patients with Barrett's esophagus who are at risk for developing an esophageal adenocarcinoma would be desirable.

A series of physiologic studies has shown that the quantity and quality of the reflux in patients with Barrett's esophagus with and without associated adenocarcinoma differs from patients with gastroesophageal reflux disease but no associated intestinal metaplasia. Reflux disease in patients with long segments of Barrett's esophagus is characterized by a markedly increased esophageal exposure to both gastric acid and duodenal contents [17, 36] (Table 1). This appears to be primarily due to a loss of lower esophageal sphincter resistance in combination with a failure of esophageal clearance function in the presence of increased basal and stimulated gastric acid secretion and increased duodenogastric reflux [33, 36].

Table 1. Lower esophageal sphincter function and esophageal acid and bile exposure in patients with intestinal metaplasia of the esophago-gastric junction and the distal esophagus (data of the Chirurgische Klinik und Poliklinik, Klinikum rechts der Isar, TU Munich)

	Control subjects (*n*=20)	EG-junction intestinal metaplasia (*n*=22)	Short segment Barrett's (*n*=28)	Long segment Barrett's (*n*=38)	Barrett's cancer (uT1) (*n*=17)
Mean LES pressure (mmHg)	12.6	11.7	7.2*	4.6*	4.8*
Mean esophageal acid exposure time on 24-h esophageal pH-monitoring (%)	2.4	3.6	8.6*	17.5*	16.9*
Mean esophageal bile exposure time on 24-h esophageal Bilitec monitoring (%)	1.2	1.9	9.9*	23.4*	25.8*

EG, esophagogastric; LES, lower esophageal sphincter; uT1, T1 category on endoscopic ultrasonography.
* $p<0.05$ versus control subjects.

Experimental data confirm the clinical observation that combined esophageal exposure to gastric acid and duodenal contents (bile acids and pancreatic enzymes) is more detrimental than isolated exposure to gastric juice or duodenal contents alone. In a variety of experimental models a combination of acid and bile reflux into the esophagus, but not acid reflux alone, induced esophageal adenocarcinoma [17, 18]. Combined reflux is thought to increase cancer risk by promoting cellular proliferation and by exposing the esophageal epithelium to potentially genotoxic gastric and intestinal contents, e.g., nitrosamines [18, 37]. This would indicate that adenocarcinoma of the distal esophagus is a direct consequence of mixed, i.e., acid and bile, reflux into the esophagus (Fig. 1) and could, at least theoretically, be prevented if the underlying chronic reflux is treated adequately and aggressively [37].

Table 1 shows data from detailed physiologic assessment of patients with various extents of intestinal metaplasia at the esophago-gastric junction or the distal esophagus. A defective lower esophageal sphincter and increased esophageal acid and bile exposure are common in patients with long and short segment Barrett's esophagus. This would indeed suggest that long and short segments of intestinal metaplasia in the distal esophagus share the same etiology, i.e., excessive reflux of gastric contents into the esophagus. In contrast, esophageal manometry and combined pH-/Bilitec monitoring did not show lower esophageal sphincter dysfunction or increased esophageal acid or bile exposure in patients who had only microscopic foci of intestinal metaplasia at or below the esophago-gastric junction (Table 1). This is in concert with other reports indicating that the prevalence and duration of heartburn as well as the prevalence of a hiatal hernia in patients with only microscopic foci of intestinal metaplasia at or below the esophago-gastric junction do not differ from control subjects [14].

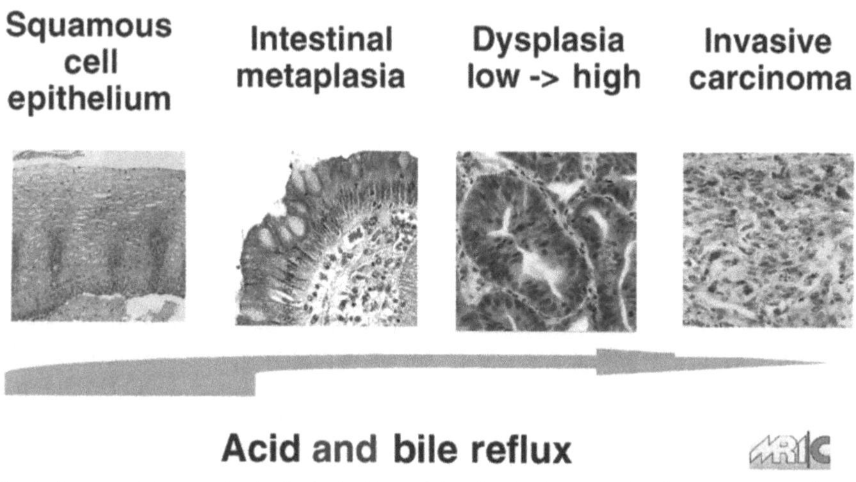

Fig. 1. Concept of the central role of mixed acid and bile reflux in the progression from squamous cell mucosa through intestinal metaplasia and dysplasia to esophageal adenocarcinoma

Helicobacter pylori, Barrett's Esophagus, and Barrett's Cancer

A series of studies has evaluated the relation between intestinal metaplasia in the distal esophagus and the presence of *Helicobacter pylori*. Most studies are consistent in the observation that *H. pylori* can infect gastric type mucosa in the distal esophagus but is unable to infect intestinal type mucosa [3]. Furthermore, in most studies there has been no difference in the prevalence of gastric *H. pylori* infection between patients with and without esophagitis and patients with long or short segments of intestinal metaplasia in the distal esophagus and control subjects [3, 13, 14, 23]. Recent reports indeed indicate that infection with CagA+ strains of *H. pylori* may even act protectively against the development of esophagitis, intestinal metaplasia, and adenocarcinoma in the distal esophagus through an as yet unknown mechanism [5, 22]. If confirmed, this observation may change our currently very liberal attitude towards *H. pylori* eradication therapy.

Studies assessing the role of *H. pylori* infection in patients with intestinal metaplasia at or below the esophago-gastric junction have so far been inconsistent [38]. Some investigators currently consider intestinal metaplasia at the esophago-gastric as a feature of *Helicobacter*-associated pan-gastritis, while others do not support this contention and relate it to inflammatory changes associated with early forms of gastroesophageal reflux disease limited to the gastric cardia.

Smoking, Alcohol, Obesity, and Barrett's Cancer

Smoking has been identified as another major risk factor for esophageal adenocarcinoma and may account for as much as 40% of cases through an early stage carcinogenic effect [12, 42]. In a Swedish population based case control study obesity was also associated with an increased risk for esophageal adenocarcinoma. In this study the adjusted odds ratio was 7.6 among persons in the highest body mass index quartile compared with persons in the lowest [6, 16]. The carcinogenic mechanism of obesity, remains to be clarified. In contrast to squamous cell esophageal cancer, there is no strong relation between alcohol consumption and adenocarcinoma of the esophagus [12].

Dysplasia and Other Markers of Malignant Degeneration of Barrett's Esophagus

Follow-up studies show that the development of Barrett's adenocarcinoma follows a multistep process in which the metaplastic epithelium sequentially develops low-grade dysplasia, high-grade dysplasia, early adenocarcinoma, and eventually invasive carcinoma [11]. Epithelial atypia in Barrett's mucosa is usually assessed according to the system devised for atypia in ulcerative colitis, namely: negative, positive, or indefinite for dysplasia [26]. One of the major challenges for the pathologist in Barrett's esophagus is the differentiation of dysplasia from reactive or regenerative epithelial changes. This is particularly difficult if erosions or ulcerations are present [11]. If there is doubt as to whether reactive and regenerative changes or dysplasia is present in a biopsy, the category atypia, indefinite for dysplasia, is appropriate and a repeat biopsy after reflux control by medical acid suppression or anti-reflux therapy should be performed.

Dysplasia in Barrett's mucosa can be detected in approximately 10% of the patients, and it develops only in the intestinal type metaplastic epithelium. The diagnostic reproducibility is not perfect, with interobserver variation for the distinction between reactive hyperplasia and low-grade dysplasia, and between high-grade dysplasia and intramucosal carcinoma [24].

Since at present, there are no clinical or histologic parameters that allow one to predict in which patients Barrett's esophagus will progress to dysplasia or adenocarcinoma [11], investigations of the molecular mechanisms associated with malignant degeneration have become a major focus of recent studies. A variety of molecular genetic changes have been correlated with the metaplasia-dysplasia-carcinoma sequence. These include alterations of tumor suppressor genes (p53, APC, FHIT, p16), growth factors (Fas, DGFR, c-erbB2), cell adhesion molecules (E-cadherin, CD44m, catenins), proteases (uPA), proliferation markers (Ki-67), and molecules involved in membrane trafficking (rab11). Most of these changes, occur late in the metaplasia-dysplasia-carcinoma sequence and can thus not be used to identify patients at risk for esophageal adenocarcinoma or as early markers of malignant deterioration [11, 19, 41].

Barrett's Esophagus: Management Issues

Treatment of Gastroesophageal Reflux in Patients with Barrett's Esophagus

Unfortunately many patients with Barrett's esophagus are unsymptomatic or have only little reflux symptomatology despite a markedly increased esophageal exposure to gastric and duodenal juice. This is believed to be due to a decreased pain sensitivity of the columnar esophageal lining. A patient presenting with Barrett's esophagus typically reports on a long history of reflux symptoms in the past with a sudden disappearance of these symptoms. This usually coincides with the appearance of the columnar lining in the distal esophagus [34].

In clinical practice the medical treatment of gastroesophageal reflux disease in patients with Barrett's esophagus matches that of patients with gastroesophageal reflux disease without Barrett's esophagus. Complete symptom eradication with proton pump inhibitors in patients with Barrett's esophagus does, however, not guarantee normalization of the intra-esophageal pH profile [21]. Rather these patients usually require much higher doses of proton pump inhibitors for normalization of the intra-esophageal acid exposure. Standard medical acid suppression therapy alone has no or only little effect on esophageal bile exposure [36] (Fig. 2a). A combination of proton pump inhibitors with prokinetic agents (e.g., cisparide) appears to be more effective in control of mixed, i.e., acid and duodenal, reflux [17].

In contrast to medical acid suppression therapy, antireflux surgery is very effective in abolishing both acid and bile reflux into the esophagus [36] (Fig. 2b). The long term control of reflux symptoms by Nissen fundoplication in patients with established Barrett's esophagus is, however, not as convincing as in reflux patients without Barrett's esophagus. The initial rate of symptom control by antireflux surgery in patients with Barrett's esophagus is in the order of 80%. Results of Nissen fundoplication in these patients, however, tend to deteriorate markedly on long-term follow-up (Table 2). Disruption of the antireflux procedure over time due to an underlying esophageal shortening and subsequent continuous tension on the fundoplication is believed to be the reason for this [9].

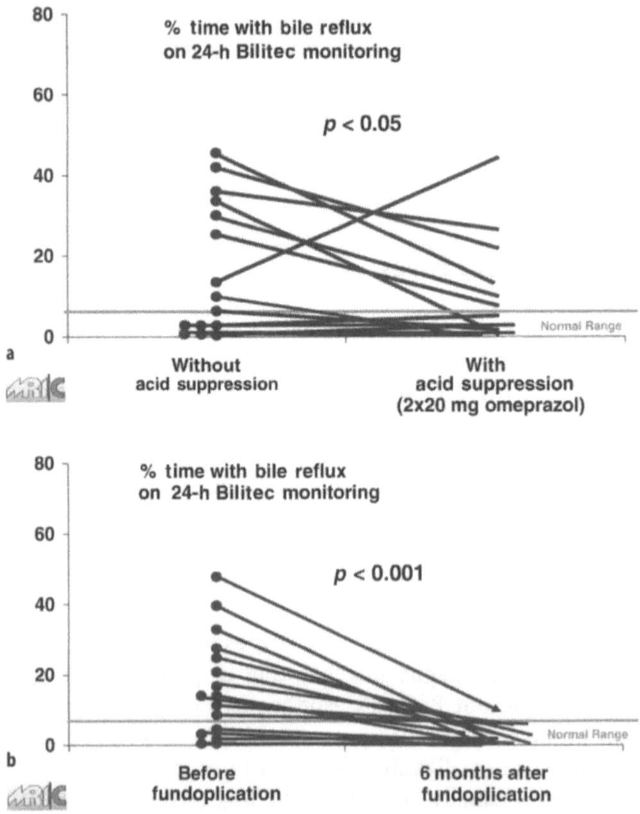

Fig. 2. Effect of standard medical acid suppression (**a**) and Nissen fundoplication (**b**) on gastroesophageal bile reflux as assessed by 24-h esophageal Bilitec monitoring

Table 2. Barrett's esophagus: symptom control by antireflux surgery

Author/Year	Fundoplications for Barrett's esophagus (*n*)	Median follow-up (years)	Excellent or good outcome (%)
DeMeester 1990	35	3	77
Williamson 1990	37	5	92
Attwood 1992	19	3	79
MacDonald 1996	113	6.5	83
Ortiz 1996	32	5	90
Cendes 1998	152	8.5	41
TU Munich 1997	82	6.5	79

Table 3. Barrett's esophagus: regression of extent after antireflux surgery

Author/Year	Fundoplications for Barrett's esophagus (*n*)	Patients with partial regression (*n*) (%)	Patients with complete regression (*n*) (%)
Wellinger 1988	39	0 (0)	0 (0)
DeMeester 1990	35	0 (0)	0 (0)
Williamson 1990	37	4 (10.8)	0 (0)
Attwood 1992	19	n.a.	2 (10.5)
Sagar 1995	56	19 (33.9)	5 (8.9)
Ortiz 1996	32	8 (25.0)	0 (0)
TU Munich 1999	82	10 (12.1)	3 (3.6)

n.a., not available.

Effect of Reflux Suppression on Extent and Malignant Potential of Barrett's Esophagus

In recent years it has been shown that medical acid suppression therapy and antireflux surgery can result in partial squamous re-epithelialization of Barrett's metaplasia [8]. However, the presence of squamous islands in a long segment with Barrett's esophagus should not be equated with regression of Barrett's esophagus or with decreased cancer risk [28]. In fact, neither complete acid suppression nor antireflux surgery will result in a predictable disappearance or regression of the extent of Barrett's esophagus (Table 3).

Similarly, there is currently no convincing evidence that either medical acid suppression or effective antireflux surgery will prevent the occurrence of dysplasia and carcinoma in patients with an established Barrett's esophagus. All series with long-term follow-up after antireflux surgery in patients with Barrett's esophagus show that carcinoma may still develop. Although it has been argued that most of these cancers appeared a relative short time period after antireflux surgery (and may have consequently already been there before the surgical procedure) or in patients with an ineffective antireflux procedure, several well-documented cases with carcinoma appearing more than

Table 4. Incidence of Barrett's carcinoma after antireflux surgery in patients with Barrett's esophagus

Author/Year	Fundoplications for Barrett's esophagus (*n*)	Patients with Barrett's cancer follow-up (*n*) (%)	Time interval between fundoplication and cancer (years)
Brand 1980	10	1 (10.0)	4
Wellinger 1988	39	2 (5.1)	3–5
Williamson 1990	37	3 (8.1)	1–10
Attwood 1992	19	1 (5.2)	n.a.
Sagar 1995	56	1 (1.7)	9
Ortiz 1996	32	1 (3.1)	n..a.
MacDonald 1996	113	3 (2.7)	1–4
Csendes 1998	152	4 (2.6)	7
TU Munich 1999	82	4 (3.6)	2, 4 and 9

n.a.; not available.

5 years after successful Nissen fundoplication have been reported in the literature (Table 4). Overall, the incidence of esophageal adenocarcinoma in patients with Barrett's esophagus who had antireflux surgery matches that of patients who had no treatment or patients who were treated medically. Patients with established Barrett's esophagus therefore need to remain under close endoscopic surveillance irrespective of the treatment.

Role of Mucosal Ablation

Endoscopic ablation of intestinal mucosa in the distal esophagus is, at least theoretically, an interesting concept to prevent the metaplasia-dysplasia-carcinoma of Barrett's esophagus. In several studies it has been shown that mucosal ablation by thermal injury, laser coagulation, or photodynamic therapy does indeed result in squamous cell re-epithelialization in an acid-free environment. A complete ablation of the entire esophageal segment with intestinal metaplasia is, however, often not possible and reoccurrence of intestinal metaplasia on long-term follow-up after successful complete ablation is frequent. Furthermore, squamous re-epithelialization may occur over an underlying glandular mucosa, thus covering up areas with malignant potential and making endoscopic surveillance impossible [39]. Esophageal adenocarcinoma thus may still occur after ablation therapy, and several such cases have already been reported. Finally, esophageal perforations and esophageal strictures requiring repeated dilatation therapy have been reported after ablation therapy [4]. Consequently, endoscopic ablation of Barrett's esophagus, although appealing, currently constitutes a potentially dangerous procedure without proven benefit for the patient.

Management of Barrett's Esophagus

Despite its high prevalence and malignant potential, many questions remain unresolved in the management of patients with Barrett's esophagus. Since neither acid suppression therapy nor antireflux surgery with or without mucosal ablation appear to reliably protect against malignant degeneration, close endoscopic surveillance with extensive biopsies is mandatory in all patients with known Barrett's esophagus of more than 3 cm in length. Esophageal adenocarcinoma carcinoma detected in patients who are under endoscopic surveillance is usually of early stage and can be cured by esophagectomy [40]. Despite the broad advocation of endoscopic surveillance in patients with known Barrett's esophagus, more than 50% of patients with esophageal adenocarcinoma, however, still have locally advanced or metastatic disease at the time of presentation [29, 34]. Whether endoscopic surveillance should also be advocated in patients with short segments of Barrett's esophagus is currently a point of controversy [27, 35].

The optimal time interval of surveillance is determined by the presence of dysplasia. In patients without dysplasia an interval of 1-2 years appears sufficient [27]. In patients with low-grade dysplasia the surveillance interval should be shortened to 3-6 months. In patients with high-grade dysplasia, an invasive cancer may already be present somewhere else in the Barrett's mucosa [27]. These patients should be referred to an expert center for immediate re-endoscopy and extensive biopsies guided by endoscopic staining or immunfluorescence techniques [25]. If invasive carcinoma can be definitely ruled out, mucosal resection may be attempted if the patient is of poor surgical risk. Most experts, however, agree that surgical resection remains the therapy of choice in patients with proven high-grade dysplasia in Barrett's esophagus [35].

References

1. Blot WJ, Devesa SS, Kneller RW, Fraumeni JF (1991) Rising incidence of adenocarcinoma of the esophagus and gastric cardia. JAMA 265:287–289
2. Blot WJ, Devesa SS, Fraumeni JF Jr (1993) Continuing climb in rates of esophageal adenocarcinoma: an update. JAMA 270:1320
3. Bowrey DJ, Williams GT, Clark GWB (1998) Interactions between Helicobacter pylori and gastroesophageal reflux disease. Dis Esophagus 11:203–209
4. Bremner CG, Demeester TR (1998) Proceedings from an international conference on ablation therapy for Barrett's mucosa. Dis Esophagus 11:1–27
5. Chow WH, Blaser MJ, Blot WJ, Gammon MD, Vaughan TL, Risch HA, Perez-Perez GI, Schoenberg JB, Stanford JL, Rotterdam H, West AB, Fraumeni JF Jr (1998) An inverse relation between cagA+ strains of Helicobacter pylori infection and risk of esophageal and gastric cardia adenocarcinoma. Cancer Res 58:588–590
6. Chow WH, Blot WJ, Vaughan TL, Risch HA, Gammon MD, Stanford JL, Dubrow R, Schoenberg JB, Mayne ST, Farrow DC, Ahsan H, West AB, Rotterdam H, Niwa S, Fraumeni JF Jr (1998) Body mass index and risk of adenocarcinomas of the esophagus and gastric cardia. J Natl Cancer Inst 90:150–155

7. Clark GWB, Smyrk TC, Burdiles P, Hoeft SF, Peters JH, Kiyabu M, Hinder RA, Bremner CG, DeMeester TR (1994) Is Barrett's metaplasia the source of adenocarcinomas of the cardia? Arch Surg 129:609–614
8. Cooper BT, Neumann CS, Cox MA, Iqbal TH (1998) Continuous treatment with omeprazole 20 mg daily for up to 6 years in Barrett's oesophagus. Aliment Pharmacol Ther 12:893–897
9. Csendes A, Braghetto I, Burdiles P, Puente G, Korn O, Diaz JC, Maluenda F (1998) Long-term results of classic antireflux surgery in 152 patients with Barrett's esophagus: clinical, radiologic, endoscopic, manometric, and acid reflux test analysis before and late after operation. Surgery 123:645–657
10. Devesa SS, Blot WJ, Fraumeni JF Jr (1998) Changing patterns in the incidence of esophageal and gastric carcinoma in the United States. Cancer 83:2049–2053
11. Flejou JF, Hainaut P, Höfler H, Keller G, Lambert R, Stein HJ, Werner M (1999) Tumours of the oesophagus/adenocarcinomas. In: WHO classification of tumours. Pathology and genetics of tumours of the digestive system (in print)
12. Gammon MD, Schoenberg JB, Ahsan H, Risch HA, Vaughan TL, Chow WH, Rotterdam H, West AB, Dubrow R, Stanford JL, Mayne ST, Farrow DC, Niwa S, Blot WJ, Fraumeni JF Jr (1997) Tobacco, alcohol, and socioeconomic status and adenocarcinomas of the esophagus and gastric cardia. J Natl Cancer Inst 89:1277–1284
13. Hackelsberger A, Gunther T, Schultze V, Manes G, Dominguez-Munoz JE, Roessner A, Malfertheimer P (1998) Intestinal metaplasia at the gastro-oesophageal junction: Helicobacter pylori gastritis or gastro-oesophageal reflux disease? Gut 43:17–21
14. Hirota WK, Loughney TM, Lazas DJ, Maydonovitch CL, Rholl V, Wong RKH (1999) Specialized intestinal metaplasia, dysplasia, and cancer of the esophagus and esophagogastric junction: Prevalence and clinical data. Gastroenterology 116:277–285
15. Lagergren JL, Bergstrom R, Lindgren A, Nyren O (1999) Symptomatic gastroesophageal reflux as a risk factor for esophageal adenocarcinoma. N Engl J Med 340:825–831
16. Lagergren J, Bergstrom R, Nyren O (1999) Association between body mass and adenocarcinoma of the esophagus and gastric cardia. Ann Intern Med 130:883–890
17. Marshall REK, Anggiansah A, Owen JW (1997) Bile in the esophagus: clinical relevance and ambulatory detection. Br J Surg 84:21–28
18. Miwa K, Hattori T, Miyazaki I (1995) Duodenogastric reflux and foregut carcinogenesis. Cancer 75:1426–1432
19. Montesano R, Hollstein M, Hainaut P (1996) Genetic alterations in esophageal cancer and their relevance to etiology and pathogenesis: a review. Int J Cancer 69:225–235
20. Nandurka S, Talley NJ (1999) Barrett's oesophagus: the long and the short of it. Am J Gastroenterol 94:30–40
21. Ouatu-Lascar R, Triadafilopoulos G (1998) Complete elimination of reflux symptoms does not guarantee normalization of intraesophageal acid reflux in patients with Barrett's esophagus. Am J Gastroenterol 93:711–716
22. Peek RM Jr, Vaezi MF, Falk GW, Goldblum JR, Perez-Perez GI, Richter JE, Blaser MJ (1999) Role of Helicobacter pylori cagA(+) strains and specific host immune responses on the development of premalignant and malignant lesions in the gastric cardia. Int J Cancer 82:520–524
23. Pereira AD, Suspiro A, Chaves P, Saraiva A, Gloria L, de Almeida JC, Leitao CN, Soares J, Mira FC (1998) Short segments of Barrett's epithelium and intestinal metaplasia in normal appearing oesophago-gastric junctions: the same or two different entities? Gut 42:659–662
24. Reid BJ, Haggitt RC, Rubin CE, Roth G, Surawicz CM, Van Belle G, Lewin K, Weinstein WM, Antonioli DA, Goldman H, MacDonald W, Owen D (1998) Observer variation in the diagnosis of dysplasia in Barrett's oesophagus. Hum Pathol 19:166–178
25. Reid BJ, Weinstein WM, Lewin KJ, Haggitt RC, Van Deventer G, Den Besten L, Rubin CE (1988) Endoscopic biopsy can detect high grade dysplasia or early adenocarcinoma in Barrett's oesophagus without grossly recognisable neoplastic lesion. Gastroenterology 94:81–90

26. Riddell RH, Goldman H, Ransohoff DF, Appelman HD, Fenoglio CM, Haggitt RC, Ahren C, Correa P, Hamilton SR, Morson BC (1983) Dysplasia in inflammatory bowel disease: standardized classification with provisional clinical applications. Hum Pathol 14:931–968
27. Sampliner RE (1998) Practice guidelines on the diagnosis, surveillance, and therapy of Barrett's esophagus. The Practice Parameters Committee of the American College of Gastroenterology. Am J Gastroenterol 93:1028–1032
28. Sharma P, Morales TG, Bhattacharyya A, Garewal HS, Sampliner RE (1998) Squamous islands in Barrett's esophagus: what lies underneath? Am J Gastroenterol 93:332–335
29. Siewert JR, Stein HJ (1997) Barrett's cancer: indications, extent and results of surgical resection. Sem Surg Oncology 13:245–252
30. Siewert JR, Stein HJ (1998) Classification of carcinoma of the oesophagogastric junction. Br J Surg 85:1457–1459
31. Spechler SJ, Goyal RK (1996) The columnar-lined esophagus, intestinal metaplasia, and Norman Barrett. Gastroenterology 110:614–621
32. Spechler SJ (1999) The role of gastric carditis in metaplasia and neoplasia at the gastroesophageal junction. Gastroenterology 117:218–228
33. Stein HJ, Hoeft S, DeMeester TR (1993) Functional foregut abnormalities in Barrett's esophagus. J Thorac Cardiovasc Surg 105:107–111
34. Stein HJ, Siewert JR (1993) Barrett's esophagus: Pathogenesis, epidemiology, functional abnormalities, malignant degeneration and surgical management. Dysphagia 8:276–288
35. Stein HJ, Panel of Experts (1996) Esophageal cancer: screening and surveillance. Results of a consensus conference. Dis Esoph 9 [Suppl 1]:3–19
36. Stein HJ, Kauer WKH, Feussner H, Siewert JR (1998) Bile reflux in benign and malignant Barrett's esophagus. Effect of medical acid suppression and fundoplication. J Gastrointest Surg 2:333–341
37. Stein HJ, Kauer WKH, Feussner H, Siewert JR (1999) Bile acids as components of the duodenogastric refluate: detection, relationship to bilirubin, mechanism of injury and clinical relevance. Hepatogastroenterology 46:66–73
38. Stein HJ, Feith M (1999) Pathogenesis of Barrett's esophagus: role of gastroesophageal reflux and helicobacter pylori. In: Peracchia A, Bonavina L (eds) Barrett's esophagus: an up-to-date. Edra, Milano, pp 17–24
39. Van Laethem JL, Cremer M, Peny MO, Delhaye M, Deviere J (1998) Eradication of Barrett's mucosa with argon plasma coagulation and acid suppression: immediate and mid term results. Gut 43:747–751
40. Van Sandick JW, van Lanschot JJB, Kuiken BW, Tytgat GNJ, Offerhaus GJA, Obertop H (1998) Impact of endoscopic biopsy surveillance of Barrett's oesophagus on pathological stage and clinical outcome of Barrett's carcinoma. Gut 43:216–222
41. Werner M, Mueller J, Walch A, Höfler H (1999) The molecular pathology of Barrett's esophagus. Histol Histopathol 14:553–559
42. Zhang ZF, Kurtz C, Marshall JR (1997) Cigarette smoking and esophageal and gastric cardia adenocarcinoma. J Natl Cancer Inst 89:1247–1249

28. Riddell RH, Goldman H, Ransohoff DF, Appelman HD, Fenoglio CM, Haggitt RC, Ahren C, Correa P, Hamilton SR, Morson BC, (1983) Dysplasia in inflammatory bowel disease: standardized classification with provisional clinical applications. Hum Pathol 14:931–968

[illegible]

New Diagnostic Methods for Esophageal Carcinoma

A. G. Bohorfoush

Department of Medicine, Division of Gastroenterology,
Medical College of Wisconsin, 9200W. Wisconsin Avenue, Milwaukee,
WI 53226, USA

Abstract

The increasingly severe problem of esophageal carcinoma on world public health merits the application of new endoscopic methods to assist in early detection and screening. Older methods, such as tissue staining, combined with magnification endoscopy, have shown promising results, while newer techniques capitalize on measurements that discriminate benign from malignant cells based on a wide array of different attributes, ranging from the molecular to the macroscopic level. Instrumentation based on laser-induced fluorescence spectroscopy, ratio fluorescence imaging, elastic scattering spectroscopy, Raman spectroscopy, and optical coherence tomography is presently being tested and compared with standard endoscopic techniques. Using pathologic interpretation of pinch biopsies as the "gold standard," these techniques have shown the ability to identify dysplastic or malignant regions of tissue that would not be visible to the unassisted endoscopist and offer increased sensitivity for detection compared to rigorous random biopsy protocols. The rapid speed of the instruments allows the provision of information to the endoscopist almost instantaneously, potentially allowing therapeutic decisions to be conducted within the confines of the same endoscopic procedure, thereby achieving gains in efficiency and reductions in overall cost. Large, multicenter trials will be necessary to determine the sensitivity and specificity of individual and combined techniques, as well as their ability to favorably influence the early detection, management, and overall outcome of this disease.

Introduction

Esophageal carcinoma is a worldwide problem with a poor prognosis if not identified at an early stage. The rising incidence of adenocarcinoma of the esophagus in particular has led to increased attention on screening individuals who are at high risk for Barrett's esophagus and following them with

Recent Results in Cancer Research, Vol. 155

surveillance examinations in order to detect premalignant changes, such as high-grade dysplasia [1]. Hence, there is a need for better diagnostic methods for detecting cancerous and precancerous changes in the esophagus so that intervention can be initiated to either prevent an incipient malignancy or cure an early cancer.

The present methods of screening for cancerous or precancerous changes primarily involves endoscopy of the esophagus, although mass screening with balloon cytology of the esophageal epithelium has also shown promise [2]. With endoscopic screening, the visual interpretation of the esophageal epithelium by the examining physician is the primary means of detection of an abnormality. While macroscopic and exophytic changes are abundantly evident to the experienced endoscopist, the microscopic changes of dysplasia are very difficult to observe, leading to the present practice of obtaining multiple random biopsies of epithelium at risk, such as Barrett's esophagus, for later interpretation by a pathologist. This approach has numerous disadvantages, such as the separation in time and space between the endoscopic examination and the histologic interpretation, the discordance of interpretation of high-grade dysplasia among pathologists [3, 4], and the need for a separate endoscopic procedure if an abnormality is detected that would require endoscopic intervention.

Efforts to improve the early detection of cancers and precancers have attempted to take advantage of the differences between normal and cancerous or precancerous tissues at the subcellular, cellular, and multicellular level [5] (Table 1). Subcellular attributes of cancer include, but are not limited to, a shift in the oxidation to reduction ratio of substances such as reduced nicotinamide adenine dinucleotide (NADH) and reduced nicotinamide adenine dinucleotide phosphate (NADPH), decrease enzyme activity (e.g., ferrochelatase), altered concentrations of certain molecules, such as nucleic acids, and the presence of abnormal proteins, such as mutant p53 or oncofetal antigens.

Cellular attributes of cancer include enlargement and hyperchromicity of cell nuclei, increased concentration of metabolic organelles such as mitochondria, Golgi apparatus, and endoplasmic reticulum, the presence of abnormal protein packages or particles, and the expression of different proteins and receptors on the cell membrane.

Multicellular attributes of cancer include the presence of disorganized epithelial orientation and architecture, changes in the epithelial surface texture and thickness, increased distance from the underlying subepithelial collagen layer, and violation of cell–cell contact inhibition, leading to invasion of nearby structures.

New Optical Technologies

There are a variety of different optical technologies that are presently under investigation to determine their effectiveness at improving the early detection and treatment of gastrointestinal cancers and precancers. Many of these have

Table 1. Attributes of cancer

Dimension	Trait	Optical method for measurement
Multicellular	Disorganized epithelial orientation and architecture	ESS, OCT
	Changes in the morphology of epithelial surface texture and thickness	ESS, LIFS, OCT
	Cell crowding, increased distance from subepithelial collagen layer	ESS, LIFS, OCT
Cellular	Enlargement and hyperchromicity of cell nucleus	ESS, OCT
	Increased concentration of metabolic organelles (e.g., Golgi apparatus, mitochondria, endoplasmic reticulum)	ESS
	Presence of abnormal protein packages or particles	ESS
Subcellular	Shift of NADH, NADPH to oxidized states by hypermetabolic cell metabolism	LIFS
	Decreased activity of ferrochelatase and/or other changes in heme synthesis	LIFS, PDD, PDT
	Altered concentration of nucleic acids and their forms (RNA, DNA), proteins, lipids, and flavins	RS
	Presence of abnormal proteins (oncofetal antigens, carbohydrate antigens, mutant p53 protein)	RS
	Increased concentration of unknown fluorophors	LIFS

ESS, elastic scattering spectroscopy; OCT, optical coherence tomography; LIFS, laser-induced fluorescence spectroscopy; PDD, photodynamic diagnosis; PDT, photodynamic therapy; RS, Raman spectroscopy; NADH, reduced nicotinamide adenine dinucleotide; NADPH, reduced nicotinamide adenine dinucleotide phosphate.

been reviewed in greater detail elsewhere [6]. These technologies approach the problem from different directions, depending upon which attributes of malignancy they are attempting to detect and measure. The imaging technologies are magnification endoscopy combined with tissue staining, or magnification chromoscopic staining (MCS), and optical coherence tomography (OCT). The spectroscopy technologies include fluorescence (laser-induced fluorescence spectroscopy, LIFS; ratio fluorescence imaging, RFI), Raman spectroscopy (RS), and elastic scattering spectroscopy (ESS). Also included within the fluorescence category is photodynamic diagnosis (PDD). Many of these technologies overlap categories, such as with RFI or PDD, which combine imaging with fluorescence.

Magnification Chromoscopic Staining

Tissue staining techniques can be employed without magnification endoscopes, but the fine details brought out by staining are much easier to appreciate at ×35 magnification [7]. Hence, staining is best performed in combination with a magnification endoscope. Tissue stains can be divided into three categories, vital or absorptive stains, reactive stains, or contrast stains

Table 2. Tissue stains

Type Vital (absorptive)	Mechanism Stains epithelial cells or cellular elements by preferential entry into cell	Stains Lugol's solution	Action stains glycogen in normal cells of the esophagus
		Methylene blue	Enters normal absorptive tissue
		Cresyl violet	Stains margins of pits on colonic mucosal surface
Reactive	Identifies cellular products	Congo red	Red to black color change at pH<3
Contrast	Highlights tissue topography	Indigo carmine	Enhances crevices and depressions, helping to discriminate polyps

[8] (Table 2). The vital stains include Lugol's solution, which stains glycogen in squamous epithelium, methylene blue, which enters normal absorptive tissue, and cresyl violet, which stains the margins of pits on colonic mucosal surfaces. The reactive stains include Congo red, which changes color from red to black at a pH of less than 3. The contrast stains include indigo carmine, which enhances the features of the tissue topography.

Optical Coherence Tomography

OCT provides micrometer-scale tomographic imaging of biologic tissues that is similar to B-mode ultrasound, except with approximately ten times greater resolution due to the use of light rather than acoustic waves [9]. Using a 1-mm probe rotated 360° on a cable, all esophageal wall layers can be visualized using a non-contact method that measures the intensity of infrared light reflected back. This information is processed into two- and three-dimensional data sets that image tissue microstructure at resolutions as high as 4 mm, rivaling that of histopathology but not requiring any physical removal of tissue. This has the distinct advantage of imaging microstructure in its native setting so that the three-dimensional characteristics of tissue abnormalities can be more accurately described [10, 11]. Presently, OCT has been tested in the gastrointestional tract in humans, but prospective trials comparing OCT with the histopathology of standard pinch biopsies for the detection of malignancies have not yet been reported.

Laser-Induced Fluorescence Endoscopy

LIFS measures the intensity of fluorescence induced by excitation wavelengths of monochromatic laser light in tissues. Known fluorophors include collagen, NADH, NADPH, flavins, tryptophan, and elastin. In malignant tissue, there may also be unknown abnormal substances which possess fluorescence. LIFS probes interrogate a small surface area with a contact tip that includes an excitation optical fiber for illumination of the tissue with the excitation wavelength and a second receptive fiber for measuring the intensity of induced fluorescence over a spectrum. This fluorescence curve is often normalized in order to amplify small spectral features and to factor out absolute intensity dependence, since tumors have such an overall weak fluorescent signal [12, 13].

An important variation of LIFS is RFI, which measures tissue autofluorescence induced by two excitation wavelengths that illuminate the entire visual endoscopic viewing field through the light bundles of the endoscope itself [14, 15]. Each pixel of the endoscope image, as acquired by the charged coupling device chip, is redisplayed in a pseudoimage after undergoing spectral fluorescent analysis. Pixels with an abnormal LIFS are displayed in a different color than those of normal tissue, leading to a compelling visual image of an island of abnormally colored dysplastic or malignant epithelium surrounded by differently colored adjacent normal epithelium. This technology is presently available for bronchoscopic screening for lung cancer and is under investigation at multiple sites for gastrointestinal applications. The distinct advantage of RFI is its ability to survey large expanses of tissue all at once instead of point by point interrogation with a probe.

Photodynamic Diagnosis

PDD combines fluorescence of an exogenously administered substance, such as porfimer sodium, or fluorescence of a substance induced by an exogenously administered precursor to that fluorophor [16]. Porfimer sodium is selectively retained for greater lengths of time in cancerous and precancerous tissue, which is extremely useful for photodynamic therapy (PDT), but which can also be used to highlight regions of undetected dysplasia or cancer in tissues that are interrogated with an LIFS device. Improvements in the detection of tissue autofluorescence have largely supplanted PDD with porfimer sodium.

Alternatively, PDD can take advantage of the accumulation within malignant cells of protoporphyrin IX (PPIX) after exposure to its precursor in the heme cycle, 5-aminolevulinic acid (5ALA) [17]. Apparently due to the relative deficiency within tumors of the enzyme ferrochelatase, PPIX cannot be metabolized as quickly as in normal tissues, leading to bright fluorescence in malignant cells with appropriate wavelength excitation. 5ALA can be taken up locally by epithelial tissues, thereby avoiding systemic administration, which is useful for both PDD and PDT [18].

Raman Spectroscopy

RS is also a probe-based technique of tissue interrogation in which the frequency shift in the illuminating wavelength of light is used to measure the vibrational and rotational frequency of the molecules within the cells of the tissue. While only a limited number of biological substances fluoresce, most biological molecules are Raman active, leading to the ability to generate much more detailed information about a tissue with distinctive spectral signatures, or biochemical fingerprints [19]. Hence, proteins, nucleic acids, nucleosomes, and cell membrane conformations can all be measured with RS. Prospective trials have been conducted with RS to detect cervical neoplasia [20], and gastrointestinal studies are under investigation as well.

Elastic Scattering Spectroscopy

ESS is also a contact probe-based technique and measures the elastic optical transport of tissue, which consists of elastic scattering and absorption. Using white light instead of laser light for excitation of tissue, the scattered light that returns to the probe is measured for its intensity across a broad spectrum (e.g., 320–800 nm), generating a unique histogram of the interrogated tissue. The scattering of light through the tissue is dependent upon the wavelength of the light and the size of the particle (the so-called Mie effect). Consequently, tissue particles such as the cell nucleus and cellular organelles scatter wavelengths that are closest to their size, i.e., on the order of 320–900 nm. ESS has been tested in a variety of organ systems, including the gastrointestinal tract, and has shown promising results [21]. Due to its ability to be used interstitially, ESS is particularly useful with needle-based probes, which can be inserted directly into a mass or solid organ, achieving the equivalent of a "smart needle." This has been used with endoscopic ultrasound-guided fine needle aspiration [22] and is undergoing testing in other solid organ systems, such as the breast and prostate.

Conclusion

The need for better detection and diagnosis of esophageal cancers is clear, and the optical technologies of the future are making rapid progress in improving the screening and surveillance of individuals at risk for these malignancies. In all likelihood, combinations of the various optical approaches to the diagnosis of neoplasia will be necessary to achieve highly reliable and reproducible results with sufficient sensitivity and specificity to permit immediate therapeutic intervention within a single endoscopic procedure [23]. The expense of these new instruments may be partially or completely offset by the savings achieved by either improved outcomes or a reduction in the number of overall procedures performed in order to prevent or cure an esophageal cancer. Prospective studies will be necessary to prove and measure the benefits gained by these new technologies.

References

1. Spechler SJ (1992) Endoscopic assessment of premalignant esophageal disorders. Gastrointest Endosc Clin North Am 2:383–394
2. Hu N et al. (1998) Quantitative fluorescence image analysis of DNA content and nuclear morphology on esophageal balloon cytology smears and subsequent development of esophageal and gastric cardia cancer in Linxian, China. Cancer Epidemiol Biomark Prevent 7(1):59–64
3. Jensen P et al (1995) Observer variability in the assessment of type and dysplasia of colorectal adenomas, analyzed using kappa statistics. Dis Colon Rectum 38:195–198
4. Melville DM et al (1989) Observer study of the grading of dysplasia in ulcerative colitis: comparison with clinical outcome. Hum Pathol 20:1008–1014
5. Naber SP (1994) Molecular pathology: detection of neoplasia. N Engl J Med 331:1508–1510
6. Bohorfoush AG (1996) Tissue spectroscopy for gastrointestinal Diseases. Endoscopy 28:372–380
7. Stevens PD (1994) Combined magnification endoscopy with chromoendoscopy for the evaluation of Barrett's esophagus. Gastrointest Endosc 40:747–749
8. Kim CY, Fleischer DE (1997) Colonic chromoscopy. A new perspective on polyps and flat adenomas. Gastrointest Clin North Am 7(3):423–437
9. Tearney GJ et al (1997) Optical biopsy in human gastrointestinal tissue using optical coherence tomography. Am J Gastroenterol 92(10):1800–1804
10. Fujimoto JG et al (1998) New technology for high-speed and high-resolution optical coherence tomography. Ann NY Acad Sci 838:95–107
11. Kobayashi K et al (1998) High resolution cross-sectional imaging of the gastrointestinal tract using optical coherence tomography: preliminary results. Gastrointest Endosc 47(6):515–523
12. Vo-Dinh T et al (1995) In vivo cancer diagnosis of the esophagus using differential normalized fluorescence (DNF) indices. Lasers Surg Med 13:23–30
13. Panjehpour M et al (1995) Spectroscopic diagnosis of esophageal cancer: new classification model, improved measurement system. Gastrointest Endosc 41:577–581
14. Lam S et al (1992) Detection of dysplasia and carcinoma in situ by ratio fluorometry. Am Rev Respir Dis 146:1458–1461
15. Lam S et al (1993) Detection of dysplasia and carcinoma-in-situ with a lung imaging fluorescence endoscope device. J Thorac Cardiovasc Surg 105:1035–1040
16. Bjorkman DJ et al (1991) Fluorescence localization of early colonic cancer in the rat by hematoporphyrin derivative. Lasers Surg Med 11:263–270
17. Bedwell J et al (1992) Fluorescence distribution and photodynamic effect of ALA-induced PP IX in the DMH rat colonic tumor model. Br J Cancer 65:818–824
18. Vonarx V et al (1997) Potential efficacy of a delta 5-aminolevulinic acid bioadhesive gel formulation for the photodynamic treatment of lesions of the gastrointestinal tract in mice. J Pharm Pharmacol 49(7):652–656
19. Mahadevan-Jensen A, Richards-Kortum R (1996) Raman spectroscopy for the detection of cancers and precancers. J Biomed Opt 1:31–70
20. van Mahade A et al (1995) Optical techniques for the diagnosis of cervical precancers: comparison of Raman and fluorescence spectroscopies. SPIE Proc 2388:110–120
21. Mourant JR et al (1995) Detection of gastrointestinal cancer by elastic scattering and absorption spectroscopies with the Los Alamos Optical Biopsy System. SPIE Proc 2387:210–217

22. Bohorfoush AG et al (1995) White light optical biopsy for detection of dysplasia or malignancy. Gastroenterology 108:A449
23. Van Dam J (1996) Laser induced fluorescence spectroscopy: somewhere over the rainbow. Gastroenterology 110:643–644

Esophageal Carcinoma: Current Staging Strategies

C. Meyenberger, A.C. Fantin

Department of Internal Medicine, Kantonsspital, CH-9007 St. Gallen, Switzerland

Abstract

A patient with suspected esophageal carcinoma represents a challenge to the treating physicians. Most patients present with an advanced stage of disease, and in the majority of cases only palliative treatment can be offered. Various treatment modalities are available, which are applied according to the TNM stage of the disease and the performance status of the patient. A precise histological diagnosis and highly accurate tumor staging of a patient with esophageal carcinoma is a prerequisite for the selection of the most suitable treatment option. Endoscopic ultrasound (EUS) has emerged as the most accurate diagnostic modality for locoregional staging. Problems in identifying early tumor stages or tumor strictures can be generally overcome by using miniprobe sonography (MPS). EUS/fine-needle aspiration biopsy (FNA) technology provides a valuable means of identifying suspicious locoregional lymph nodes. Patients with a proximal tumor (trachea bifurcation) should undergo bronchoscopy to rule out infiltration of the tracheobronchial system. Ultrasound (US), computed tomography (CT), and possibly magnetic resonance imaging (MRI) are the diagnostic tools of choice for extended tumor staging. After excluding extended tumor stage and severe concomitant diseases, diagnostic laparoscopy with intra-abdominal ultrasound should be performed in patients with adenocarcinoma of the esophagus prior to esophagectomy. Intra-abdominal metastases which can be missed preoperatively in some cases have to be ruled out in order to avoid unnecessary surgery.

General Considerations

The majority of patients with esophageal carcinoma (EC) present with advanced-stage disease at the time of diagnosis. However, it is necessary to detect esophageal cancer at an early stage in order to be able to improve the dismal prognosis of this disease. Selecting the appropriate treatment based on accurate staging is of paramount importance [1, 2].

Recent Results in Cancer Research, Vol. 155

Although there has been some improvement in the overall 5-year survival rate, the overall 5-year survival is generally reported to be only 10%–15%. The prognosis of esophageal carcinoma is closely related to the tumor stage. In one series of resected tumors, the 5-year survival rate in patients with early cancers (T1 and T2) was 41% versus 13% in patients with more advanced cancers (T3 and T4) [3]. When the patients were stratified according to lymph node infiltration, those without lymph node involvement had a 5-year survival rate exceeding 40% compared to only 19% of patients with malignant mediastinal lymph nodes. Preoperative staging should identify the subset of patients with invasive unresectable carcinoma (T4) or distant metastases who have a poor outcome, irrespective of the type of treatment, with a median survival of only 3–8 months [4].

Impact of Staging on Treatment

In esophageal carcinoma, pretherapeutic staging is most important, since different treatment modalities have to be chosen according to the tumor stage and localization. The possibility of complete tumor resection (R0) is mainly based on the anatomical topography and the tumor stage according to the TNM classification (Appendix) with respect to the local tumor invasion (T stage), the regional lymphatic spread (N stage), and the absence or presence of distant metastases (M stage). In tumors above the tracheal bifurcation, an R0 resection is possible only in early stages of disease (T1, T2) without infiltration of vital neighboring structures, such as the tracheobronchial system.

Management of early tumors involves not only curative surgery, but also endoscopic therapy, such as mucosectomy, photodynamic therapy, and laser ablation in selected patients [5]. For advanced disease, a multimodal approach is indicated combining neoadjuvant radiochemotherapy with surgery or a primary palliative procedure (endoluminal stent, laser ablation) in poor candidates for surgery and in patients with extended disease [6–8].

Distant metastases at presentation are a poor prognostic sign, usually obviating any surgical approach with a median survival of only several months. In a recent series of 838 patients with esophageal carcinoma, 18% of all patients already had distant metastases at presentation [9].

Diagnosis and Staging

After establishing the diagnosis of esophageal cancer, distant metastases precluding curative surgery should be ruled out by computed tomography (CT) and/or abdominal sonography (Fig. 1). If distant metastases are found, locoregional staging is not relevant to the treatment strategy. If distant metastases can be ruled out, endoscopic ultrasound (EUS) is the most accurate technique for determining the depth of tumor invasion and the involvement of local lymph nodes. EUS with miniprobes (miniprobe sonography, MPS),

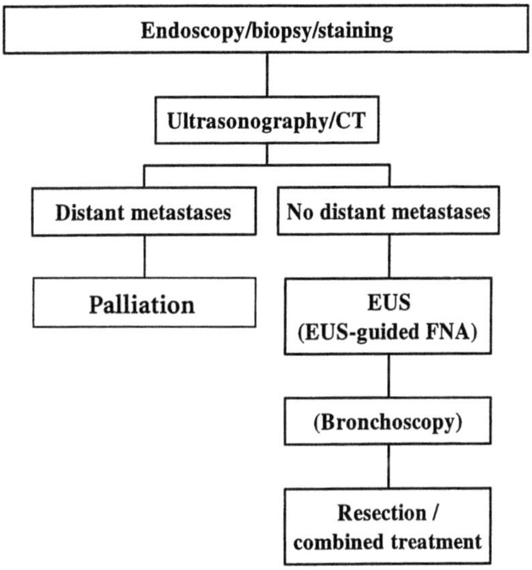

Fig. 1. Staging algorithm. Endoscopy can be performed in combination with endoscopic ultrasound (*EUS*) using a miniprobe (MPS) as a single-step procedure for both diagnosis and locoregional tumor staging. Bronchoscopy should be performed in suprabifurcal located esophageal cancer. Laparoscopy and intraoperative ultrasound are recommended for adenocarcinoma of the distal esophagus. *CT*, computed tomography; *FNA*, fine-needle aspiration biopsy

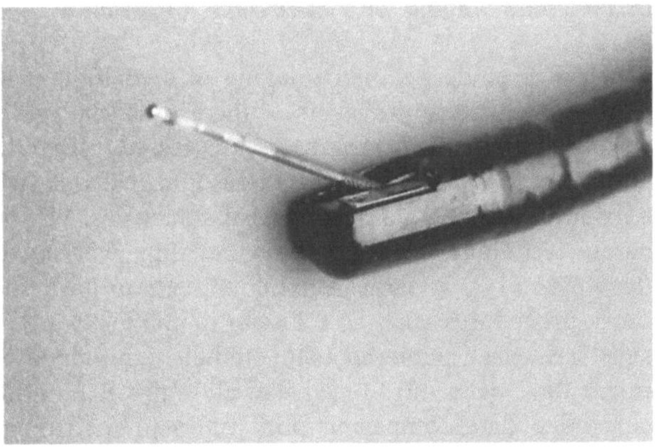

Fig. 2. Instrument used in miniprobe sonography (MPS) which can be introduced through the working channel of a conventional endoscope

which can be introduced into the working channel of a normal endoscope (Fig. 2), might change the proposed algorithm. MPS can be performed at the same time as the diagnostic endoscopy is undertaken to provide a single-step procedure for both diagnosis and local staging. Furthermore, MPS is used in tumor strictures that cannot be passed using a conventional echo endoscope, thus avoiding prior dilatation. A new linear scanning echo endoscope with EUS-guided fine-needle aspiration biopsy (FNA) is reported to improve the diagnostic accuracy of malignant lymph nodes.

Diagnosis

The diagnosis and assessment of the longitudinal extension of esophageal carcinoma are established by endoscopy with biopsy. In addition to conventional histopathological typing and grading, it might be useful to determine molecular markers in the future [10]. Barium studies are used to evaluate the morphology of the tumor.

Extended Staging

After histological diagnosis in a patient with esophageal cancer, extended tumor staging with abdominal sonography and/or CT should follow. In certain circumstances, magnetic resonance imaging (MRI) with contrast medium or positron emission tomography (PET) might be preferred to investigate liver metastases. Distant metastases of esophageal cancer preclude surgical options and make the patient a candidate for palliative treatment.

Locoregional Staging with Endoscopic Ultrasound

EUS can provide detailed imaging of a malignant esophageal tumor and its relationship within the layers of the esophageal wall (Fig. 3). The depth of invasion through the layers can be assessed using the four tumor stages. T1 and T2 tumors are limited to the esophageal wall, whereas T3 and T4 tumors have infiltrated the paraesophageal structures. EUS is at present the most accurate technique for local tumor staging, with an overall accuracy of more than 80% [11]. A large number of papers have shown its superiority over other procedures such as CT scan or MRI [12–16]. Most of the reported results have been achieved using radial scanning EUS. Recently, linear instruments have been introduced that allow for EUS-guided FNA. Some surgically controlled data comparing both types of instruments are available that report similar staging results [17].

The overall accuracy for assessing the T and N stage and for predicting resectability is reported to be as high as 82%–90%, 70%–90%, and 80%–92%, respectively [18]. There are several limitations of EUS for staging esophageal carcinoma. For various reasons, depending on the tumor stage, the accuracy of locoregional staging varies between 80% and 92%. The staging of T2 lesions is most difficult. Overstaging is usually due to peritumoral inflammation, and understaging is related to microscopic invasion beneath the spatial resolution of EUS [19]. EUS currently cannot precisely differentiate between tumors limited to the mucosa (T1m stage) and those infiltrating the submu-

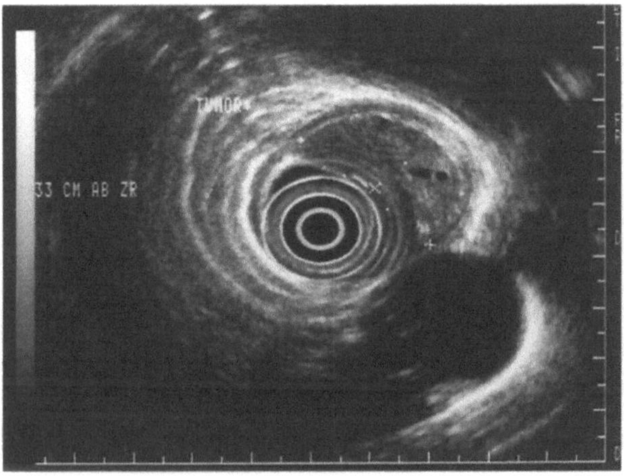

Fig. 3. Esophageal cancer confined to the first low-echo layer of the esophageal wall (T1 tumor)

cosa (T1sm stage), which is a prerequisite for local endoscopic therapy. T1m tumors without infiltration of the lamina muscularis mucosae present with malignant lymph node involvement in only 5%–9% of patients, whereas T1sm tumors are found to have metastasized in 30%–40% [20, 21]. The use of EUS using a miniprobe (MPS) working with higher ultrasound frequencies can overcome these limitations. In a series of 54 patients with superficial esophageal carcinoma, an overall accuracy of 75% was found for tumor staging [22]. The accuracy in differentiating between cancer limited to the mucosa and that extending to the submucosal layer was 94% of all cases.

The accuracy rate for staging more advanced tumor stages using the classical TNM classification is more than 80% for T3 and T4 carcinomas [12]. In a recent paper, muscularis propria disruption and irregular mass borders, the two classical criteria for tumors invading through the muscularis propria (T3 or T4), were found to have low accuracy rates of only 44% and 50%, whereas the maximal tumor thickness (overall or extraesophageal) of the esophageal mass was found to have a much higher accuracy of 79% and 87% in predicting a T3 or T4 tumor [17]. It can be concluded from this study that the measurement of the maximal thickness of a malignant esophageal mass by EUS is a more objective parameter that can accurately predict extraesophageal extension and that this criterion is superior to the more subjective, operator-dependent criteria usually used for T staging.

Diagnosis of local tumor invasion into the tracheobronchial system is a crucial point and often underestimated by EUS. CT and bronchoscopy are reported to achieve higher accuracy rates in predicting tracheobronchial infiltration [23].

Complete tumor staging, especially the evaluation of periesophageal and celiac lymph nodes, may be limited by tumor stenosis that cannot be passed by a conventional echo endoscope (Fig. 4). The average percentage of impassable tumor strictures is about 30% [12, 24]. Patients with impassable steno-

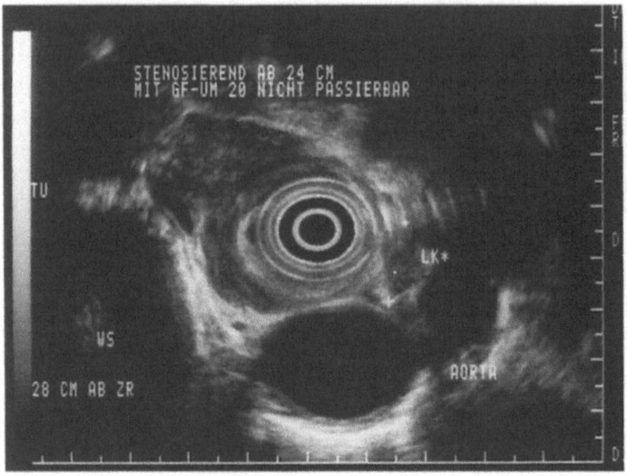

Fig. 4. Impassable stenosing esophageal cancer with a locoregional malignant lymph node

sis are likely to have advanced disease in over 75% of cases [24, 25]. Dilatation of tumor strictures before endosonographic examination may lead to esophageal perforation in up to 24% [24]. It is recommended that the risk of perforation can be reduced by gradual dilatation instead of a single dilatation session. A recent paper suggested that the risk of perforation may have been overestimated in the past [25]. At present, there are two new methods to overcome this problem: the use of a small-diameter blind ultrasonic probe (esophagoprobe), which can be introduced via a guidewire, or the radial or linear ultrasonic miniprobe (MPS) mentioned above, which can be introduced through the working channel of a conventional endoscope. These miniprobes usually use higher frequencies ranging from 7.5 to 20 MHz. Only few surgically controlled data have been published so far comparing the staging accuracy of the different small-diameter ultrasonic systems. A very recent paper including 53 patients with stenosing esophageal cancer evaluated the use of ultrasonic miniprobes compared with conventional EUS [26]. The overall accuracy rates for depth of tumor infiltration staging were 62% for the combination of conventional EUS with an esophagoprobe and 86.8% for MPS. The staging accuracy rates were 88.2%, 95.7%, and 100% for T2, T3, and T4 stages, respectively. Using miniprobes, the staging for T2 tumors was reported to significantly exceed that of the other echo endoscopes. However, overstaging was reported in four of seven T1 tumors, demonstrating the still unresolved problem in this setting. The celiac lymph nodes were able to be assessed in 89.5% of cases. Accuracy rates for assessing malignant locoregional lymph node involvement were similar in the three different systems. The major advantage of using MPS is the combination of endoscopic and endosonographic evaluation in the same session, resulting in a single-step procedure that is more convenient for patients and also lowers costs.

The diagnosis of lymph node metastases is of paramount prognostic importance. Patients with locoregional lymph node metastases have a poor prognosis, while over 40% of patients without malignant lymph nodes are still alive after 5 years [3]. The overall accuracy rate for diagnosing malignant lymph nodes is reported to be as high as 77%, ranging from 50% to 90% [27]. Comparable results are achieved with MPS [27]. There are no strict objective endosonographic criteria to differentiate between a malignant and a benign lymph node. EUS-guided FNA of suspicious lymph nodes using a linear scanning echo endoscope may improve diagnostic accuracy. In a multicenter prospective evaluation of EUS-guided FNA for primary diagnosis, staging, and follow-up examinations in 457 patients with 554 lesions, the technique was reported to be safe with a very low rate of severe nonfatal complications of only 0.5%. Sensitivity, specificity, and accuracy for lymph nodes was 92%, 93%, and 92%, respectively [28]. The same accuracy rate of ultrasonography-guided aspiration biopsy in diagnosing metastatic lymph nodes was achieved in 52 patients with non-small-lung cancer [29].

It is generally accepted that performing endosonography requires substantial experience to achieve the high staging accuracy rates reported in the literature. In 1994, the working party for the Tenth World Congress of Gastroenterology in Los Angeles recommended that a minimum of 50 examinations should have been performed to attain sufficient skill in staging esophageal cancer [30]. In a recent paper concerning 71 patients with surgically controlled data, overall staging accuracy in patients investigated by an experienced endosonographer was 83% compared to only 58% in those who were examined by a less experienced physician. This study showed a definitive learning curve for endosonographic T staging of esophageal cancer. Acceptable results could only be achieved after 100 examinations.

EUS also provides important information on localization (tracheal bifurcation), longitudinal extension, and submucosal infiltration of the tumor, which is often underestimated by endoscopy [31]. Although EUS is generally thought to be limited to locoregional staging, distant lymph node metastases of the celiac axis, which are considered as distant metastases (M1), and of the left liver lobe can be explored by EUS. However, the few data dealing with this problem have shown low accuracy rates of only 60%–68% [12].

Locoregional Staging with Computed Tomography Compared with Endoscopic Ultrasound

A large number of papers have compared the staging accuracy of EUS with CT and have shown its superiority, especially for locoregional staging. CT scan should nonetheless be considered complementary and should be combined with EUS to diagnose extraesophageal tumor infiltration into mediastinal organs and distant metastases. Locoregional staging with CT depicts an aortic or tracheobronchial infiltration with an accuracy of 55%–96% and 74%–97%, respectively [32]. Regional and abdominal lymph nodes are diagnosed with an accuracy of 51%–70% and 83%–87% [23].

As previously discussed, EUS is superior to CT in differentiating between T1 and T2 tumors and in assessing locoregional lymph nodes. However, CT is known to be superior to EUS in detecting malignant abdominal lymph nodes and malignant infiltration of the trachea and in diagnosing distant metastases.

Extended Staging: Laparoscopy Versus Computed Tomography/Ultrasound

Preoperative laparoscopic examination is an important additional diagnostic method for extended staging in potentially resectable adenocarcinoma of the esophagogastric junction. In a study of 145 patients with adenocarcinoma of the esophagogastric region (n=110) and squamous cell-type carcinoma (n=35), a prospective comparison of laparoscopy and combined imaging (CT and abdominal ultrasound) was carried out. Metastatic disease outside the potential field of resection was diagnosed in 27% of all patients. The sensitivities of laparoscopy and the combined imaging for the diagnosis of metastases were 77% and 38%, respectively. Peritoneal metastases were detected preoperatively in 23 of 24 patients by laparoscopy (sensitivity, 96%), whereas they were only detected in five patients using combined imaging (sensitivity, 21%) [33]. In addition to its superiority in diagnosing peritoneal metastases in adenocarcinoma of the esophagogastric junction, laparoscopy has the advantage of facilitating biopsy under direct vision and of being able to be combined with laparoscopic ultrasound. It is important to note that, in several studies, additional intra-abdominal pathologies were found in 19%–53% using laparoscopy combined with intraoperative laparoscopic ultrasound [33–35].

Appendix: TNM Classification for Esophageal Carcinoma [36]

T *Primary tumor*
- TX Primary tumor cannot be assessed
- T0 No evidence of primary tumor
- T1 Tumor invades lamina propria or mucosa
- T2 Tumor invades muscularis propria
- T3 Tumor invades adventitia
- T4 Tumor invades adjacent structures

N *Regional lymph nodes*
- NX Regional lymph nodes cannot be assessed
- N0 No regional lymph node metastases
- N1 Regional lymph node metastases

M *Distant metastases*
- MX Distant metastases cannot be assessed
- M0 No distant metastases
- M1 Distant metastases

For tumors of lower thoracic esophagus:
M1a Metastases in celiac lymph nodes
M1b Other distant metastases
For tumors of upper thoracic esophagus:
M1a Metastases in cervical lymph nodes
M1b Other metastases
For tumors of midthoracic esophagus:
M1a Not applicable
M1b Nonregional lymph node or other distant metastases

References

1. Peters JH et al (1994) Selection of patients for curative or palliative resection of esophageal cancer based on preoperative endoscopic ultrasonography. Arch Surg 129:534–539
2. Hoelscher AH et al (1995) Staging concepts for gastrointestinal malignancies: the importance of preoperative locoregional T and N staging. Gastrointest Endosc Clin North Am 5:534–539
3. Siewert JR, Hoelscher AH, Dittler HJ (1990) Preoperative staging and risk analysis in esophageal carcinoma. Hepatogastroenterology 37:382–387
4. Hiele M et al (1997) Relation between endoscopic ultrasound and outcome of patients with tumors of the esophagus or esophagogastric junction. Gastrointest Endosc 45:381–386
5. Lightdale CJ (1996) Diagnosis, staging, and cure of early gastrointestinal cancer. Gastrointest Endosc 44:95–96
6. Walsh TN et al (1996) A comparison of multimodal therapy and surgery for esophageal adenocarcinoma. N Engl J Med 335:462–467
7. Bosset JF et al (1997) Chemoradiotherapy followed by surgery compared with surgery alone in squamous-cell cancer of the esophagus. N Eng J Med 337:161–171
8. Chak A et al (1995) Prognosis of esophageal cancers preoperatively staged to be locally invasive (T4) by endoscopic ultrasound (EUS): a multicenter retrospective cohort study. Gastrointest Endosc 42:501–506
9. Quint et al (1995) Incidence and distribution of distant metastases from newly diagnosed esophageal carcinoma. Cancer 76:1120–1127
10. Lightdale CJ (1996) Diagnosis of esophagogastric tumors. Endoscopy 28:22–26
11. Caletti GC (1998) Endoscopic ultrasonography. Digestion 59:509–529
12. Rösch T (1995) Endosonographic staging of esophageal cancer: a review of literature results. Gastrointest Endosc Clin North Am 5:537–547
13. Greenberg J et al (1994) Computed tomography or endoscopic ultrasonography in preoperative staging of gastric and esophageal tumors. Surgery 116:696–702
14. Botet JF et al (1991) Preoperative staging of esophageal cancer: comparison of endoscopic US and dynamic CT. Radiology 181:419–25
15. Dittler HJ et al (1993) Role of endoscopic ultrasonography in esophageal carcinoma. Endoscopy 25:156–161
16. Koch J et al (1994) Staging esophageal cancer: computed tomography, magnetic resonance imaging and endoscopic ultrasound. Semin Roentgenol 29:364–372
17. Brugge WR et al (1997) Endoscopic staging criteria for esophageal cancer. Gastrointest Endosc 45:147–152
18. Rösch et al (1992) Local staging and assessment of resectability in carcinoma of the esophagus, stomach, and duodenum by endoscopic ultrasonography. Gastrointest Endosc 38:460–467
19. Grimm et al (1993) Endosonography for preoperative locoregional staging of esophageal and gastric cancer. Endoscopy 25:224–230

20. Ide H et al (1994) Esophageal squamous cell carcinoma: pathology an progress. World J Surg 18:321–330
21. Yoshi Y et al (1993) Mucosal carcinoma of the esophagus with vessel invasion and lymph node metastases: an analysis of cases collected from three institutions. Gastrointest Endosc 35:2516–2524
22. Murata Y et al (1996) Small ultrasonic probes for determination of the depth of superficial esophageal cancer. Gastroinest Endosc 44:23–28
23. Saunders HS et al (1997) Esophageal cancer: radiologic staging. Radiol Clin North Am 35:281–294
24. Van Dam J et al (1993) High-grade malignant stricture is predictive of esophageal tumor stage. Cancer 71:2910–2917
25. Kallimanis GE (1995) Endoscopic ultrasound (EUS) for staging esophageal cancer, with or without dilatation, is clinically important and safe. Gastrointest Endosc 41:540–546
26. Menzel et al (1999) Preoperative staging of esophageal carcinoma: miniprobe sonography versus conventional endoscopic ultrasound in a prospective histopathologically verified study. Endoscopy 31:291–297
27. Wiersema MJ (1994) Endosonography. In: Cotton PB et al (eds) Annual of gastrointestinal endoscopy 1994. Current Science, London, pp 133–148
28. Wiersema MJ et al (1997) Endosonography-guided fine-needle aspiration biopsy: diagnostic accuracy and complication assessment. Gastroenterology 112:1087–1095
29. Gress FG et al (1997) Endoscopic ultrasonography, fine-needle aspiration biopsy guided by endoscopic ultrasonography, and computed tomography in the preoperative staging of non-small-cell lung cancer: a comparison study. The assessment of mediastinal lymph nodes in lung malignancies. Ann Intern Med 127:604–612
30. Caletti GC et al (1994) Endoscopic ultrasonography (EUS): a summary of the conclusions of the working party for the Tenth World Congress of Gastroenterology, Los Angeles, California October, 1994. Am J Gastroenterol 89 [Suppl]:5138–5143
31. Natsugoe S et al (1996) Assessment of tumor invasion of the distal esophagus in carcinoma of the cardia using endoscopic ultrasonography. Endoscopy 28:750–755
32. O'Brien MGO et al (1995) A prospective comparison of laparoscopy and imaging in the staging of esophagogastric cancer before surgery. Am J Gastroenterol 90:2191–2194
33. Hermann K (1996) Intraoperative ultrasound in gastrointestinal cancer. An analysis of 272 patients. Hepatogastroenterology 43(9):565–570
34. Rau B et al (1996) Laparoscopic lymph node assessment in pretherapeutic staging of gastric and esophageal cancer. Recent Results Cancer Res 142:209–215
35. Hunerbein M et al (1998) The role of staging laparoscopy for multimodal therapy of gastrointestinal cancer. Surg Endosc 12:921–925
36. UICC (1997) TNM classification for esophageal cancer, 5th edn.

What's New in Imaging?

New Magnetic Resonance Imaging of Esophageal Cancer Using an Endoluminal Surface Coil and Antibody-Coated Magnetite Particles

S. Ozawa[1], Y. Imai[2], T. Suwa[1], M. Kitajima[1]

[1]Departments of Surgery and [2]Radiology School of Medicine, Keio University, 35 Shinanomachi, Shinjuku-ku, Tokyo, 160-8582 Japan

Abstract

An endoluminal surface coil: Esophageal cancer was studied by high resolution magnetic resonance imaging (MRI) to determine the histopathologic basis for signal intensity in these lesions and to determine the potential of this modality for evaluating the depth of cancer invasion. In a basic study, 14 tumors were examined with a 1.5-T superconductive MR system using a surface coil. The esophageal wall could be differentiated into four layers on the T1-weighted images and seven layers on the T2-weighted images. The signal intensity of the tumor varied from low to intermediate on the T1- and T2-weighted images. The submucosal layer is important in evaluating cancer invasion on the T2-weighted images. In a clinical study, 30 patients with esophageal cancer were examined with a 1.5-T superconductive MR system using an endoluminal surface coil. In terms of depth of cancer invasion, the accuracy rate of MRI using the endoluminal surface coil was 83%. In conclusion, MRI with an endoluminal surface coil will be a useful examination for esophageal cancer in the future.

Antibody-coated magnetite particles: A highly specific and effective MRI contrast agent was prepared by coating superparamagnetite particles with monoclonal antibodies (MAbs) directed against epidermal growth factor receptors (EGFRs), which are overexpressed in esophageal squamous cell carcinoma. The agent was shown to have EGFR-specific MRI contrast capacity in vivo in athymic rats bearing TE8 or H69 tumors. Immunospecific MRI using magnetite particles coated with MAbs against EGFR seems to be useful in the diagnosis of squamous cell carcinoma of the esophagus.

An Endoluminal Surface Coil

Introduction

Esophageal cancer is one of the most malignant tumors known and is hard to treat. Accurate staging is necessary to select appropriate therapy. Although

Recent Results in Cancer Research, Vol. 155

computed tomography (CT) and endoscopic ultrasonography (EUS) are useful examinations for staging esophageal cancer [1], each entails certain problems. CT does not provide good resolution of the esophageal wall, and is not useful for evaluating tumor invasion of the wall. EUS can provide better resolution of the esophageal wall and tumor invasion than CT, but it usually provides only transverse sections, and further analysis of tumor signals is limited. On the other hand, MRI can provide images in any direction, that is, transverse sections, sagittal sections, or coronal sections, and enables further signal analysis to evaluate tumor quality. It seems to have great potential for staging esophageal tumors. We examined esophageal cancers by high resolution MRI to determine the histopathologic basis for signal intensity in these lesions and to determine the potential of this modality in evaluating the depth of cancer invasion.

Materials and Methods

Basic study

Fourteen tumors were examined with a 1.5-T superconductive MR system using a surface coil (Signa; GE Medical Systems). Seven of the tumors were pT1, one was pT2, and six were pT3. All specimens were imaged after fixation. All images were obtained with T1-weighted images by spin echo (TR/TE 400–560, 12–17 ms) and T2-weighted images by fast spin echo (TR/TE 2000–4000, 96–114 ms).

The image area was blocked and embedded in paraffin, and sections were cut and stained with hematoxylin-eosin. The MRI findings were compared with the histologic interpretations.

Clinical Study

Thirty patients with esophageal cancer were examined with a 1.5-T superconductive MR system using an endoluminal surface coil specially manufac-

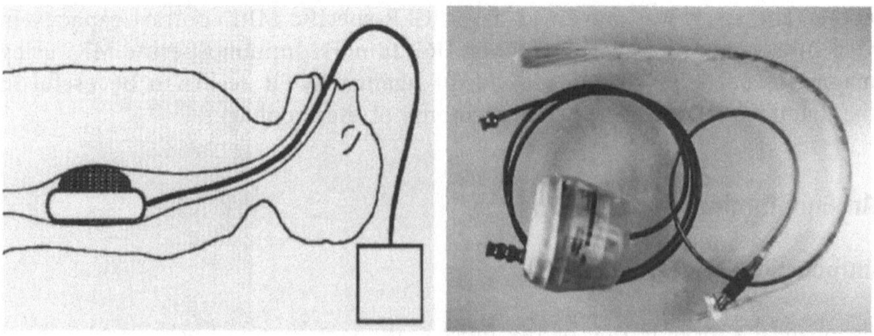

Fig. 1. An endoluminal surface coil was inserted into the esophagus through the mouth

tured by Imai (Fig. 1). The coil was inserted into the esophagus through the mouth under local superficial anesthesia, and the top balloon was inflated to open the endoluminal coil. Section thickness was 5 mm. To minimize motion artifacts, peripheral gating was utilized on the T1- and T2-weighted images and the respiratory compensation method on the T1-weighted images. The MRI findings were compared with the histologic interpretations.

Results

Basic study

On the T1-weighted images, the esophageal wall could be differentiated into four layers (Fig. 2):

1. The epithelium, the lamina propria mucosa, and the muscularis mucosa (high to intermediate signal intensity)
2. The submucosa (low intensity)
3. The muscularis propria (intermediate intensity)
4. The periesophageal fat (high intensity)

On the T2-weighted images, the esophageal wall was differentiated into seven layers:

1. The epithelium (intermediate intensity)

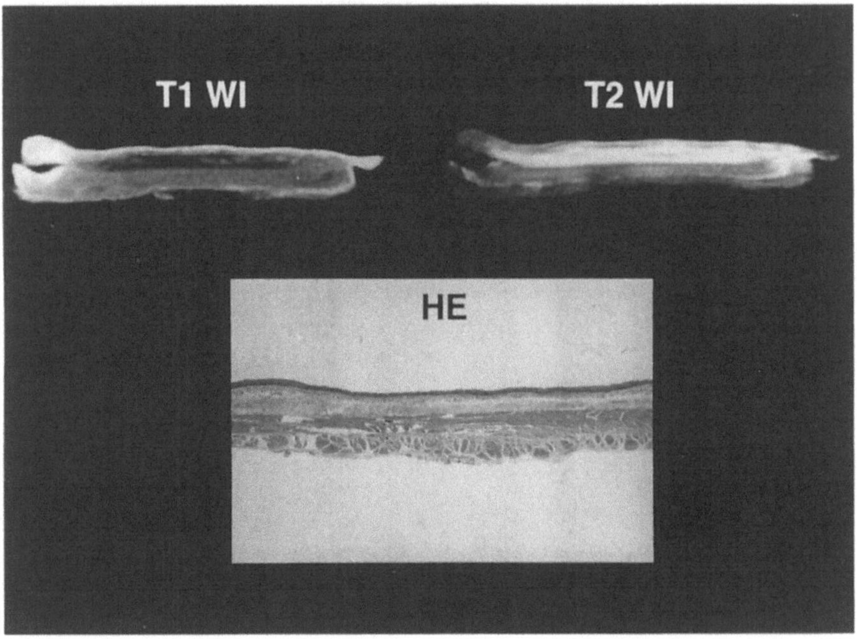

Fig. 2. Normal esophageal wall. *T1WI*, T1-weighted image; *T2WI*, T2-weighted image; *HE*, microscopic section stained with hematoxylin-eosin

2. The lamina propria mucosa and the muscularis mucosa (low intensity)
3. The submucosa (high intensity)
4. The inner, circular muscularis propria (low intensity)
5. An intermuscular structure (intermediate intensity)
6. The outer, longitudinal muscularis propria (low intensity)
7. The subadventitia structures (high intensity)

The submucosa seems to be an important landmark in the esophageal wall on T2-weighted images. The visualization of normal laminar structure of the esophageal wall was much better on the T2-weighted images than on the T1-weighted images. These findings indicated the same results as the in vitro study of colorectal tumors [2].

T1 cancer was detectable on both T1- and T2-weighted images, but tumor invasion of the submucosa was much more clearly seen on the latter (Fig. 3). The tumor showed intermediate signal intensity on both T1- and T2-weighted images.

T2 cancer was detectable only on the T2-weighted images (Fig. 4). The tumor margin could be accurately traced in the muscularis propria. T3 cancer was revealed on the T2-weighted image as interruption of the hypointense muscle layer (Fig. 5).

The signal intensities of the layers of the esophagus on the T1- and T2-weighted images are summarized in Table 1. The submucosal layer is impor-

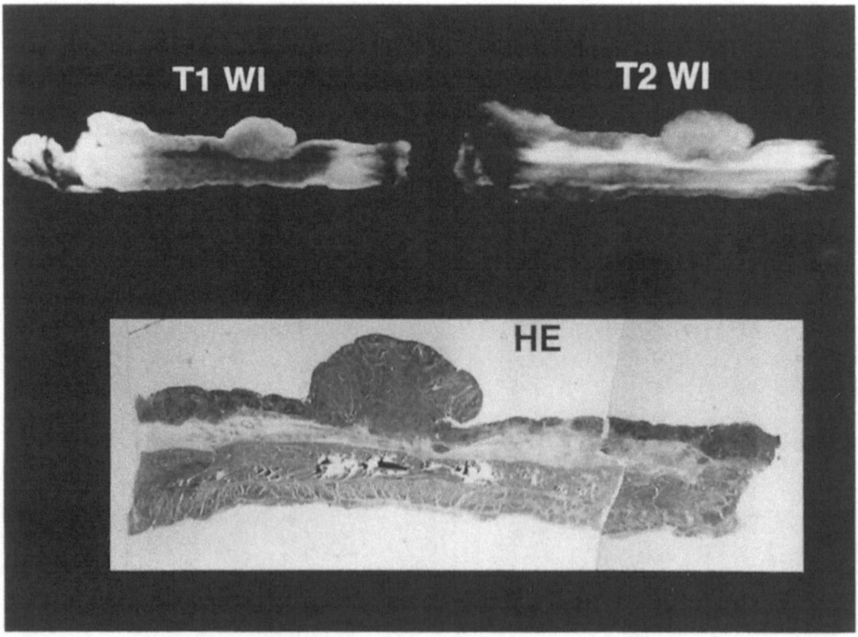

Fig. 3. pT1 cancer of the esophagus. *T1WI*, T1-weighted image; *T2WI*, T2-weighted image; *HE*; microscopic section stained with hematoxylin-eosin

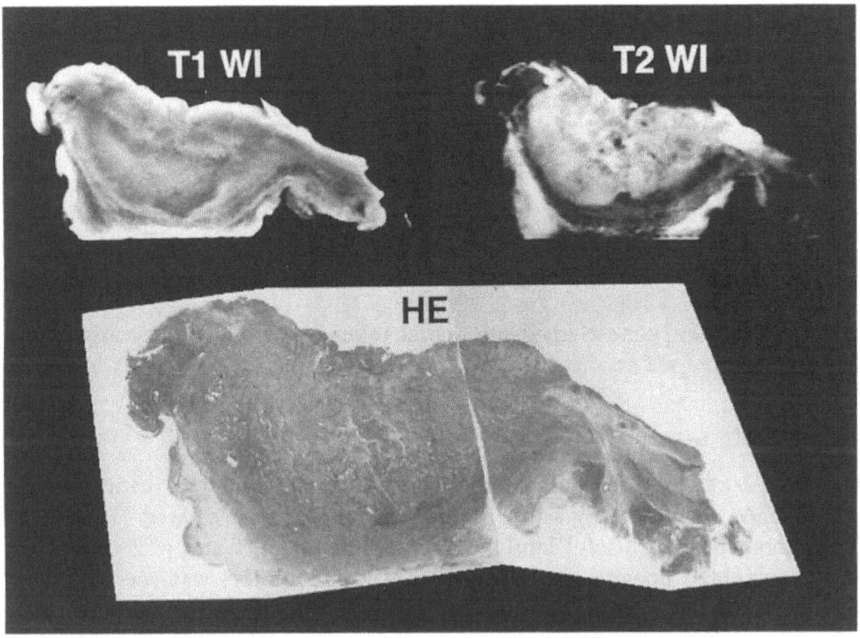

Fig. 4. pT2 cancer of the esophagus. *T1WI*, T1-weighted image; *T2WI*, T2-weighted image; *HE*, microscopic section stained with hematoxylin-eosin

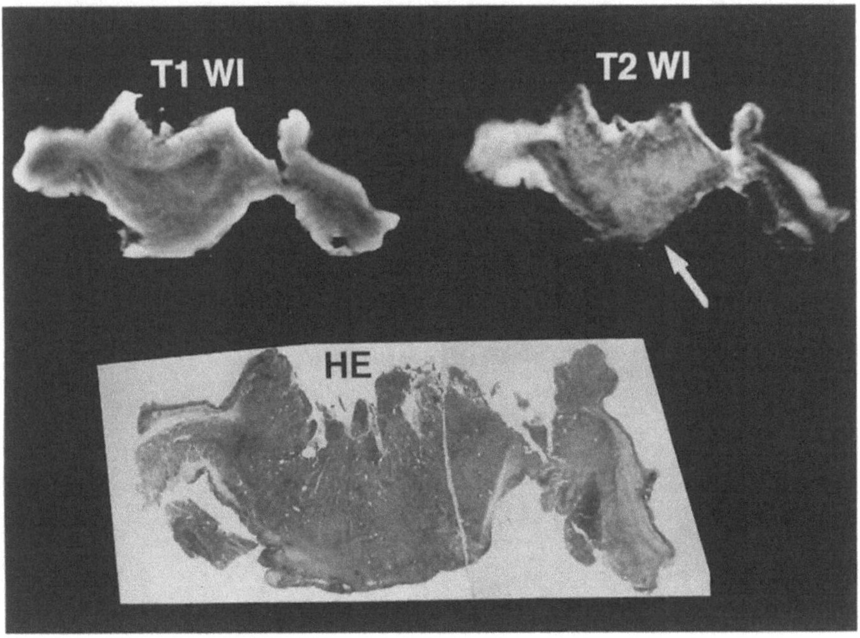

Fig. 5. pT3 cancer of the esophagus. *T1WI*, T1-weighted image; *T2WI*, T2-weighted image. *HE*, Microscopic section stained with hematoxylin-eosin

Table 1. Signal intensities of layers of the esophagus on T1- and T2-weighted images

Structure	Signal intensity	
	T1-weighted	T2-weighted
Epithelium	High	Intermediate
Propria mucosa and muscularis mucosa	Intermediate	Low
Submucosa	Low (~intermediate)	High
Muscularis propria	Low (~intermediate)	Intermediate (~low)
Tumor	Intermediate (~low)	Intermediate (~low)

tant in evaluating cancer invasion. Signal intensity of the tumor varied from low to intermediate on the T1- and T2-weighted images.

Clinical study

On the T2-weighted images, tumors, including pT1 and pT2 cancers, were well-imaged and their invasion of the wall could be evaluated (Figs. 6, 7). The submucosa is a useful landmark for evaluating pT1 and pT2 cancer. On the T1-weighted images, the outer margin of pT3 tumors was seen as an interruption of the high signal intensity layer, that is, the outer adipose tissue (Fig. 8).

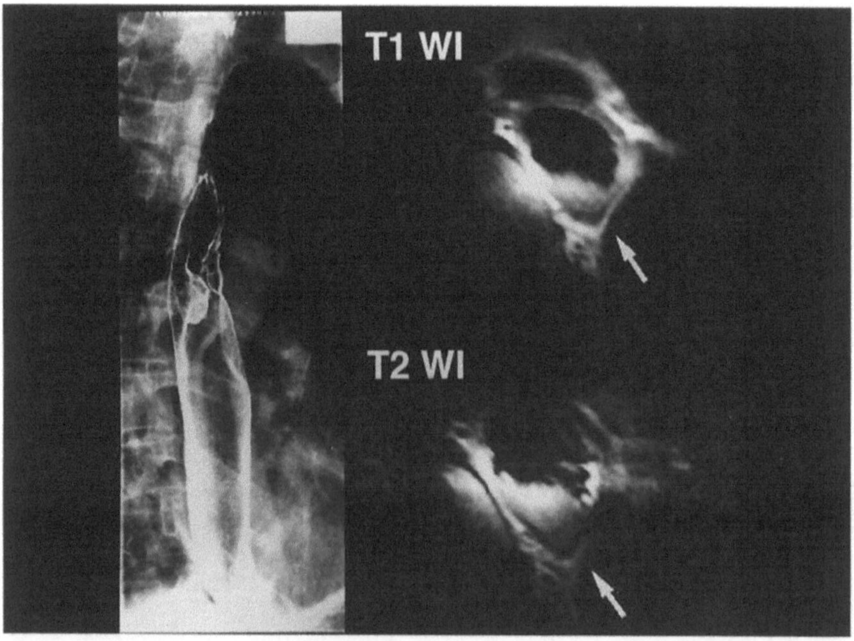

Fig. 6. pT1 cancer of the esophagus. Barium X-ray of the tumor (*left*). *Arrows* indicate the tumor. *T1WI*, T1-weighted image; *T2WI*, T2-weighted image

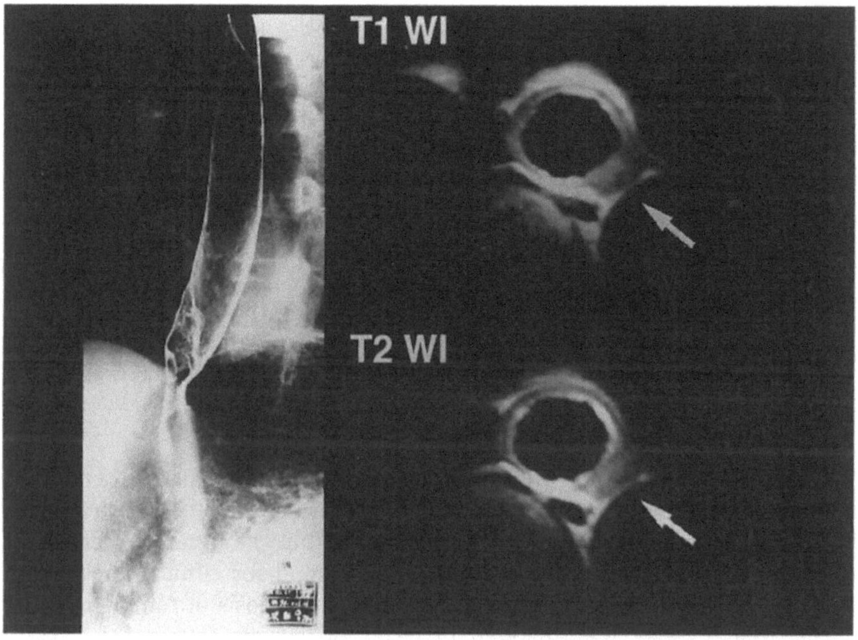

Fig. 7. pT2 cancer of the esophagus. Barium X-ray of the tumor (*left*). *Arrows* indicate the tumor. *T1WI*, T1-weighted image; *T2WI*, T2-weighted image

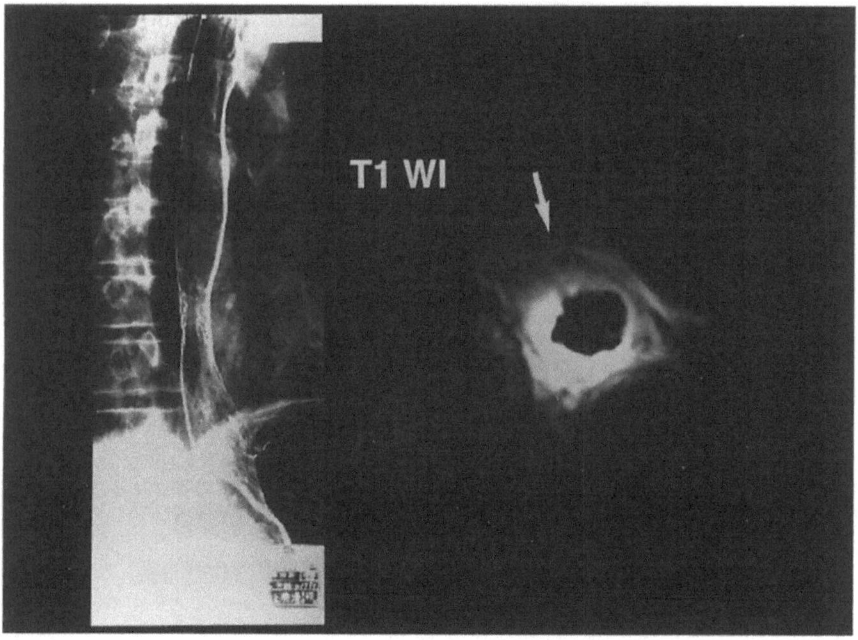

Fig. 8. pT3 cancer of the esophagus. Barium X-ray of the tumor (*left*). *Arrow* indicates the tumor. *T1WI*, T1-weighted image

Table 2. Correlation between pathological findings and the findings on MRI using an endoluminal surface coil

MRI findings	Pathological findings				
	pT1a	pT1b	pT2	pT3	Total
T1	3	8			11
T2		5	3		8
T3				11	11
Total	3	13	3	11	30

Accuracy rate: 25/30=83%)
pT1a, tumor invades the lamina propria mucosa; pT1b, tumor invades the submucosa.

Correlations between the MR images using the endoluminal surface coil and the pathological findings are shown in Table 2. Five of the 30 cases were overdiagnosed in terms of depth of cancer invasion, but the other 25 were diagnosed accurately. The accuracy rate of 83% is good for clinical application. Body coil MRI, on the other hand, did not allow diagnosis of tumor invasion.

The accuracy rate was analyzed in terms of various factors [3] (Fig. 9). The rates were almost the same for tumor location, but the tumor type of advanced tumors was more accurately diagnosed with the endoluminal surface coil. The rates were almost the same for histopathological grading and growth pattern. Accuracy depended on the shape and size of the tumor.

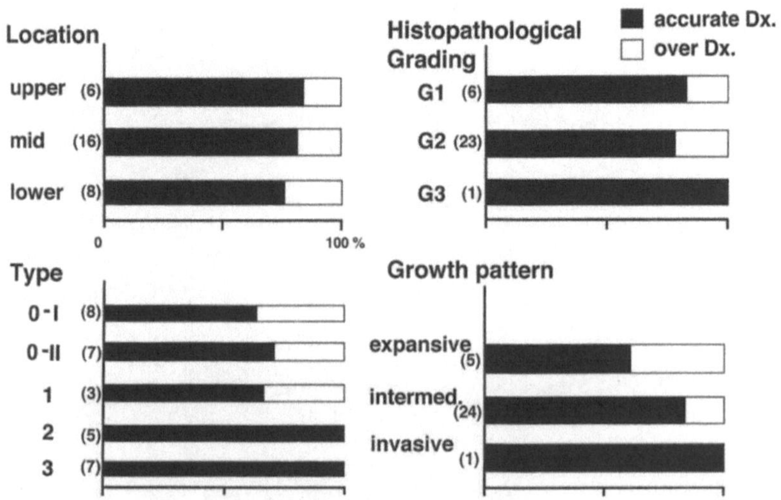

Fig. 9. Accuracy rates for evaluating tumor invasion by MR imaging with an endoluminal surface coil. *0-I*, superficial and protruding type; *0-II*, superficial and flat type; *1*, protruding type; *2*, ulcerative and localized type; *3*, ulcerative and infiltrative type

Discussion

MRI with the surface coil yielded good resolution of the esophageal wall and squamous cell carcinoma. The submucosa is a useful landmark for evaluating tumor invasion of the submucosa (pT1) and the muscularis propria (pT2), since it is visualized as high signal intensity on the T2-weighted images because of the presence of loose connective tissue, capillary vessels, and lymphatic channels. Periesophageal adipose tissue is helpful in evaluating tumor invasion of the outer structure of the esophagus (pT3), because adipose tissue is seen as high signal intensity on T1-weighted images.

Ability to diagnose tumor invasion by MRI using an endoluminal surface coil is much better than by CT but still is poorer than by EUS. In the basic study, MRI was capable of demonstrating mucosal cancer that had reached a certain thickness, but not in the clinical study. Visualization of lesions located in the lower third of the thoracic esophagus is easily influenced by the heartbeat, which adversely affects MRI because of motion artifacts, and imaging time is still longer than required for CT or EUS. These problems could be overcome by future advances in technology.

The advantage of MRI over EUS is broad visualization beyond the trachea and bronchi. Lymph nodes in the upper mediastinum are frequently involved by metastasis and should be examined closely. Although EUS cannot visualize lymph nodes beyond these airways, lymph nodes surrounded by adipose tissue are easily detected on MR images.

In the clinical study, the accuracy rate of evaluating T factor by MRI with the endoluminal coil was 83%, almost the same as by EUS in our institution, and tumors larger than pT1 can be evaluated. MRI with an endorectal surface coil has been used for clinical staging of prostate and vaginal cancer [4, 5], and MRI with an endoluminal surface coil will be applied to the staging of esophageal cancer as well.

In summary, cancer invasion limited to the esophageal wall was well-evaluated on the T2-weighted images, because the submucosal layer showed high signal intensity. Cancer invasion of periesophageal adipose tissue and lymph node metastasis were evaluated on the T1-weighted images, because the adipose tissue displayed high signal intensity. We therefore conclude that MRI with an endoluminal surface coil will be a useful examination for esophageal cancer in the future.

Antibody-Coated Magnetite Particles

Introduction

High levels of epidermal growth factor receptor (EGFR) expression are frequently observed in esophageal squamous cell carcinomas, and high EGFR levels have been reported to be a significant prognostic indicator for this tumor [6, 7]. It therefore seemed reasonable to detect EGFR as a marker of esophageal squamous cell carcinoma as a means of diagnosing tumors with greater malignant potential. The development of a noninvasive method of detecting EGFR would clearly be of great clinical significance. The decisive advantage of MRI over scintiphotography is higher spatial resolution, and the characteristics of tissues can be ascertained by measuring changes in relaxation times (T1 or T2) after the administration of magnetic agents coated with monoclonal antibodies (MAbs). Tissues that overexpress EGFR, such as metastatic lesions of squamous cell carcinomas, would be expected to show relaxation time changes after the injection of magnetic agents coated with anti-EGFR MAbs. Ferromagnetic particles exhibit marked relaxivity and in recent years have been used to improve the diagnostic capacity of MRI for liver and bone marrow malignancies, splenic lymphomas, and lymph nodal involvement, both primary and metastatic [8]. Theoretically, it is possible to achieve tumor contrast with MRI by using ferromagnetic particles coated with MAbs targeting a specific tumor antigen. As yet, however, satisfactory results have not been obtained, mainly because of the limited number of target sites. In this study, ferromagnetic particles approximately 10 nm in diameter were used. The particles were coated with anti-EGFR MAbs. Particle size was measured with a photon spectrometer, and the immunoreactivity and the relaxivity of the coated particles were confirmed to be maintained in vitro. In addition, in vivo studies were conducted to determine whether the magnetic particles coated with anti-EGFR MAbs might serve as contrast media for MRI. An athymic rat model with implanted squamous cell carcinoma was used.

Materials and Methods

Six-week-old female athymic rats (F344/N Jcl-rnu) were obtained from Clea Japan Inc (Tokyo, Japan). MAbs against the human EGF Receptor (528) were purified from ascitic fluid produced by intraperitoneally inoculating BALB/c mice with 5×10^6 hybridoma 528 cells. TE8 cells established from human squamous cell carcinoma of the esophagus were kindly provided by Dr. Nishihira (Tohoku University, Miyagi, Japan). H69 human small-cell lung cancer cells were obtained from Dr. Shimosato (National Cancer Research Institute, Tokyo, Japan). TE8 cells had elevated numbers of EGFRs (5×10^5 /cell), while H69 cells had only undetectable EGFR levels. We used TE8 cells as EGFR hyperexpressing cells and H69 cells as a negative control in this study.

Lignosite FML, an aqueous colloidal solution of a ferromagnetic iron lignosulfonate having characteristic magnetic properties (Georgia Pacific Corp., Atlanta, Ga., USA), was used. The average size of the particles was about 10 nm in diameter. MAb-coated magnetite particles (528-Fe) were prepared as previously described, with some modifications [9]. Lignosite FML was diluted to a concentration of 21.0 mgFe/ml with 10 mM HEPES buffer, pH 7.4, and this solution (1.5 ml) was added to 1.0 ml of MAb solution (2.5 mg protein/ml in 10 mM HEPES buffer, pH 7.4). The mixture was sonicated on ice three times for 1 min, at 30 s intervals, at 30 W output power using a Sonifier 250 machine (Branson, Danbury, Conn., USA). The resulting solution was layered on top of a 10 mM HEPES buffer, pH 7.4, 20 mg/ml BSA (bovine serum albumin), 30% glycerol solution, and centrifuged at 300,000 *g* for 12 min to separate particle-bound MAb from particle-free MAb. In addition to its stabilizing effect, BSA was needed to saturate additional binding sites. After centrifugation, the pellet was washed twice with 10 mM HEPES buffer, pH 7.4, and then sonicated for 30 s at 20 W to dissolve it in the same buffer. Measurement of the protein concentration of the washing solution showed that about 60% of the initially added antibody was associated with the magnetite particles. In this preparation, 1.5 mg of MAb was bound to about 30 mgFe of magnetite particles.

TE8 (2×10^7 cells in 1 ml of DMEM) or H69 cells (2×10^7 cells in 1 ml of RPMI medium 1640) were implanted into the muscle of athymic rats. After 3 weeks, the tumors reached sizes ranging from 15 to 30 mm in diameter. When the tumors reached about 20 mm in diameter, the rats were intravenously injected with 528-Fe or ns-Fe (1.5 ml of a solution containing 4 mgFe/ml). MRI was performed before and 40 h after injection with 528-Fe or ns-Fe. The athymic rats were anesthetized by intraperitoneal injection of sodium pentobarbital (60 mg/kg) (Dynabot, Osaka, Japan). The intensity of the tumor before and after injection was compared at the same slice. MRI was performed by the spin-echo technique (TR=500, 1000, 1500, or 2000 ms, TE=30, 60, 90, or 120 ms), and the T1 and T2 of tumor and muscle were calculated from the signal data at various TRs and TEs.

Results

528-Fe was injected intravenously into athymic rats that had previously been implanted with TE8 cells. The MRI of TE8 tumor-bearing rats before and 40 h after injection of 528-Fe are shown in Fig. 10. The TE8 tumor was contrasted to low intensity after 528-Fe injection. The T2 of the tumor decreased after 528-Fe injection, and TE8 tumor contrast persisted until about 5 days after the 528-Fe injection. On the other hand, the T1 of the tumor and the T1 and T2 of muscle lesions did not change greatly after injection. In a control study, the rats were injected with ns-Fe and MRI was performed. The T1 and T2 of TE8 tumor did not change greatly after the ns-Fe injection. These experiments were also performed using H69-bearing rats, and the results of 528-Fe injection are shown in Fig. 11. All experiments were performed on five rats in each group, and the T1 and T2 of the tumors are shown in Fig. 12.

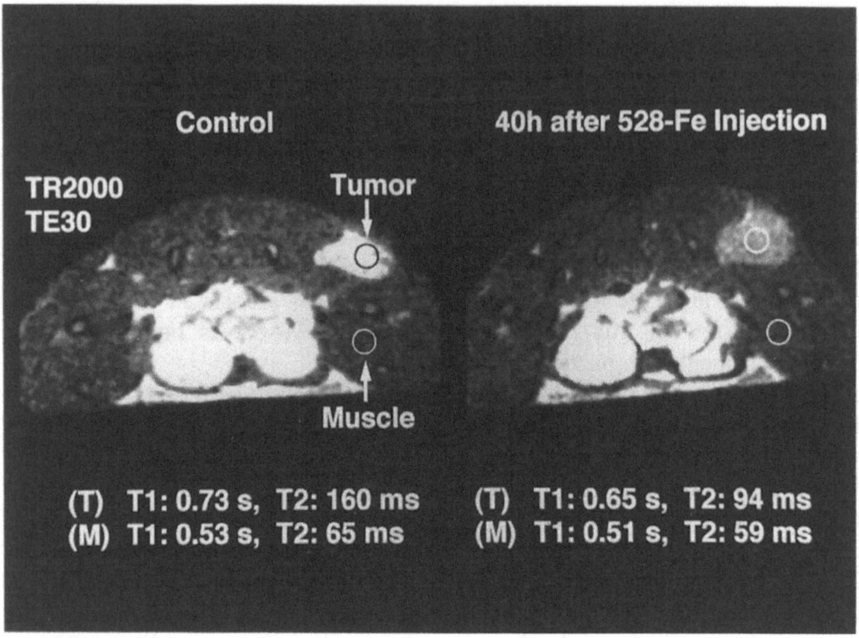

Fig. 10. MRI at TR 2000 ms and TE 30 ms of an athymic rat bearing a TE8 tumor. The *left* image is before 528-Fe injection, and the *right* image shows the same slice 40 h after 528-Fe injection. The image 40 h after injection showed lower intensity than before injection. T1 and T2 were calculated from the signal intensity of the area in the *open circles*. T2 of the tumor was 160 ms before injection and 94 ms 40 h after injection and had decreased about 40%. *T*, tumor; *M*, muscle

Discussion

Our findings indicate the feasibility of specific MRI of esophageal squamous cell carcinoma with MAbs against EGFR. We succeeded because of the very small size of the magnetite particles coated with MAbs, their superparamagnetic characteristics, and their retained immunoreactivity.

Physiologically, the permeability of the capillary wall can be understood in terms of one or two pore systems of different pore size and density. The most widely accepted concept is that there are two pore sizes, small (9 nm) and large (50–70 nm) [10, 11]. A contrast agent must cross the capillary wall before it can bind to tumor cells. Thus, maximum particle diameter is limited by the size of capillary pores, which have an approximate diameter of 50 nm. In other papers, the upper limit of particle size is said to be 50 nm [12]. Since particles larger than 20 nm would be recognized by the mononuclear phagocytic system of the lymph nodes, the size of contrast agents should be no more than 20 nm. The particle size of contrast agents should be chosen with a view to avoiding scavenging by reticuloendothelial system (RES) cells and to having enough large cores acquiring large magnetic moments. The size of the antibody-coated magnetite particles prepared in this study was measured by photon cor-

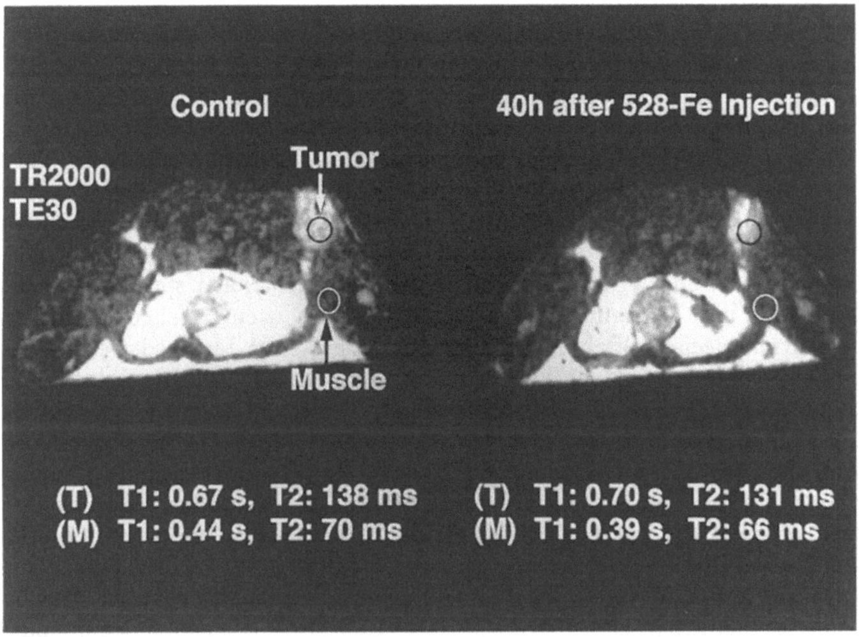

Fig. 11. MRI at TR 2000 ms and TE 30 ms of an athymic rat bearing an EGFR-deficient H69 tumor. T2 of the tumor was 138 ms before 528-Fe injection and 131 ms 40 h after 528-Fe injection. The change was not significant

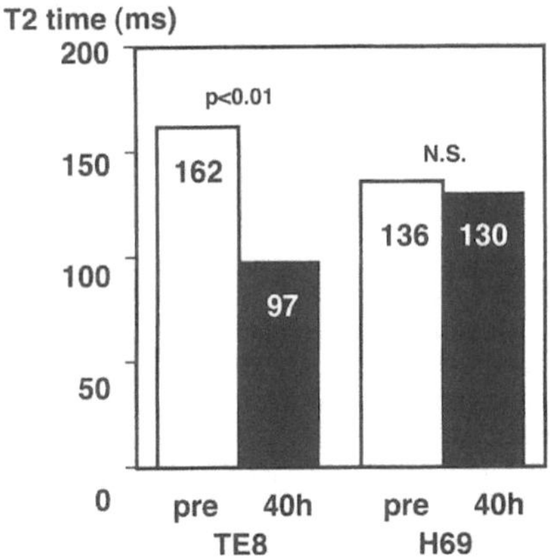

Fig. 12. T2 of TE8 tumors and H69 tumors before and 40 h after 528-Fe injection. All values are means obtained in five experiments. *By Student's *t*-test, the T2 of TE8 40 h after 528-Fe injection was shorter than before 528-Fe injection ($p<0.01$)

relation spectroscopy and found to be 13.2 nm. This is smaller than the size of the capillary pores and the size of objects that can be recognized by the cells of the RES. The value 13.2 nm was not completely accurate, since determination of their true diameter by photon correlation spectroscopy was difficult. Assessment of the extent of scavenging by the RES in progress.

Our findings in this study show that magnetite coated with anti-EGFR MAbs can be used successfully for tumor-specific MRI in a rat model bearing esophageal sqamous cell carcinomas. Until now, there has been no specific diagnostic method for squamous cell carcinoma, and this immunospecific MRI has the possibility of becoming a new diagnostic method for squamous cell carcinoma. The concept of immunospecific MRI can be applied to other molecules related to cancer. Rapid advances in MAb technology have made it possible to produce MAbs against almost any antigen that can be purified. Many cell surface receptors are usually heterogeneously distributed throughout the body, and an immunospecific contrast agent for a specific receptor population may be useful. Such agents may be very useful in checking for recurrence, especially after the primary tumor has been removed, because its antigenic nature would be known and a fairly immunospecific agent could be produced. Toxicity is also an important problem in regard to the clinical use of magnetite particles. The short-term toxicity of magnetite is quite low, with the LD50 in rats being 400 mg/kg [13]. However, investigators studying pulmonary function have reported that 10% of 2.8 μm magnetite particles remain in the lungs 1 year after a single dose [14]. Further information on the storage and toxicity of magnetite are needed before it can be used clinically.

In conclusion, we succeeded in obtaining an adequate MRI contrast effect by using magnetite particles coated with anti-EGFR MAbs in an athymic rat model bearing esophageal sqamous cell carcinoma, and this immunospecific MRI has the possibility of becoming a new diagnostic method for squamous cell carcinoma. Further studies directed at clinical application seem clearly warranted.

These two topics were based mainly on studies performed in our laboratories [15, 16].

References

1. Holscher AH, Dittler HJ, Siewert JR (1994) Staging of squamous esophageal cancer: accuracy and value. World J Surg 18:312–320
2. Imai Y, Kressel HY, Saul SH, Chao PH et al (1990) Colorectal tumors: an in vitro study of high-resolution MR imaging. Radiology 177:695–701
3. Japanese Society for Esophageal Disease. Guide lines for the clinical and pathologic studies on carcinoma of the esophagus, 8th edn
4. Schnall MD, Imai Y, Tomaszewski J et al (1991) Prostate cancer: local staging with endorectal surface coil MR imaging. Radiology 178:797–802
5. Corn BW, Lanciano RM, Rosenblum N et al (1995) Improved treatment planning for the Syed-Neblett template using endorectal coil magnetic resonance and intraoperative (laparotomy/laparoscopy) guidance: a new integrated technique for hysterectomized women with vaginal tumors. Gynecol Oncol 56:255–261
6. Ozawa S, Ueda M, Ando N et al (1987) High incidence of EGF receptor hyperproduction in esophageal squamous cell carcinomas. Int J Cancer 39:333–337
7. Ozawa S, Ueda M, Ando N et al (1989) Prognostic significance of epidermal growth factor receptor in esophageal squamous cell carcinomas. Cancer 63:2169–2173
8. Vogl TJ, Hammerstingl R, Schwarz W et al (1996) Magnetic resonance imaging of focal liver lesions. Comparison of the superparamagnetic iron oxide resovist versus gadolinium-DTPA in the same patient. Invest Radiol 31:696–708

9. Cerdan S, Lotscher H, Kunnecke B et al (1989) Monoclonal antibody-coated magnetite particles as contrast agents in magnetic resonance of tumors. Magn Reson Med 12:151–163
10. Weissleder R, Elizondo G, Wittenberg J et al (1990) Ultrasmall superparamagnetic iron oxide: characterization of a new class of contrast agents for MR imaging. Radiology 175:489–493
11. Renkin E, Curry F (1982) Endothelial permeability: pathways and modulations. Ann N Y Acad Sci 401:248–259
12. Tiefenauer LX, Kuhne G, Andres RY (1993) Antibody magnetite nanoparticles: in vitro characterization of a potential tumor-specific contrast agent for magnetic resonance imaging. Bioconjug Chem 4:347–352
13. Renshaw PF, Owen CS, Evans AE et al (1986) Immunospecific NMR contrast agents. Magn Reson Imaging 4:351–357
14. Cohen D, Arai SF, Brain JD (1979) Smoking impairs long-term dust clearance from the lung. Science 204:514–516
15. Ozawa S, Imai Y, Ando N et al (1996) High-resolution magnetic resonance imaging of esophageal cancer using an endoluminal surface coil. In: Peracchia A et al (eds) Recent advances in diseases of the esophagus. Monduzzi, Bologna, pp 165–175
16. Suwa T, Ozawa S, Ueda M et al (1997) Magnetic resonance imaging of squamous cell carcinoma using magnetite particle coated with anti-epidermal growth factor receptor antibody. Int J Cancer 75:626–634

Risk Analysis in Esophageal Surgery

H. Bartels, H. J. Stein, J. R. Siewert

Chirurgische Klinik und Poliklinik, Klinikum rechts der Isar
der Technischen Universität München, Ismaninger Straße 22, 81675 München,
Germany

Abstract

The postoperative mortality after esophagectomy still remains a major factor influencing the prognosis of esophageal cancer and largely depends on the patient's preoperative physiological status.

A composite scoring system was developed to predict the risk of esophagectomy, based on quantitative assessment of preoperatively available physiological parameters. The scoring system was reviewed retrospectively on operated patients and evaluated prospectively in two subsequent patient groups.

An initial retrospective multivariate analysis of 432 esophagectomy patients identified a compromised general status ($p = 0.001$) and poor cardiac ($p < 0.001$), hepatic ($p < 0.05$), and respiratory ($p < 0.05$) functions as independent predictors of a fatal postoperative course. Based on the relative risks associated with individual impaired organ functions – general status 3.6, cardiac function 2.8, hepatic function 2.1, pulmonary function 1.7 – a composite risk score was established. A prospective study in 121 patients confirmed that this composite scoring system provides better identification of high-risk patients than does any of the individual parameters alone. Including this composite score into the process of patient selection and choice of procedure resulted in a decrease of postoperative mortality from 9.4% (52/553) to 1.2% (4/323) ($p = 0.001$).

The risk of death after esophagectomy for esophageal cancer can be objectively assessed prior to surgery and quantified by a composite risk score. This score provides a useful tool in refining the criteria of patient selection for resection and choice of procedure, and markedly reduces postoperative mortality when applied prospectively.

Introduction

Despite recent advances in other therapeutic modalities, surgical resection provides the only chance of cure for patients with esophageal carcinoma. Esophagectomy therefore remains the therapeutic mainstay in patients with potentially resectable esophageal cancer. The morbidity and mortality asso-

Recent Results in Cancer Research, Vol. 155

ciated with esophagectomy are, however, substantial. In a recent series, the main mortality rate from esophagectomy for cancer was 13%, regardless of the surgical approach [1], and, even in experienced centers, the postoperative mortality rate ranged between 5% and 10% in the western world [1].

Several analyses have shown that, after standardization of surgical resection and reconstruction techniques, the postoperative course and postoperative mortality largely depend on the patient's preoperative risk situation [2, 3]. Therefore, a better understanding of preoperative risk factors might be one approach to reduce mortality in surgical treatment. A reduction in postoperative mortality can only be achieved by strict selection of patients with adequate physiological reserves to withstand an extended surgical procedure and a potentially prolonged and complicated postoperative course [4].

The aim of preoperative risk analysis is to reduce postoperative morbidity and mortality by identifying compromised organ functions which can be improved by preoperative measures and problem-oriented postoperative therapy. Ideally, therefore, preoperative risk assessment influences timing of the surgical procedure, choice of surgical approach, and postoperative management. Identification of relevant pre-existing disorders that may influence postoperative course is an essential requisite of risk analysis [5].

Unfortunately, none of the currently available risk-scoring systems are applicable to the specific problems associated with esophagectomy and reconstruction [6]. Therefore, most surgeons rely on patients' "impressions" and their own experience rather than objective parameters in patient selection for esophagectomy. Nevertheless, in a recent conference of the International Society for Diseases of the Oesophagus held in August 1995 in Milan, all of the participating experts agreed on the importance of objective preoperative risk analysis to improve the outcome of surgical resection for esophageal cancer [6].

In the present study, we tried to develop a composite scoring system which allows prediction of the risk of esophagectomy for cancer based on objective, preoperative physiological parameters. We addressed three specific questions:

1. Can a detailed preoperative assessment identify individual physiological parameters, i.e., risk factors, that correlate with the postoperative course?
2. Can the risk of postoperative mortality after esophagectomy be predicted using a score based on individual, preoperative physiological parameters?
3. Can the clinical use of such a scoring system reduce mortality from esophagectomy?

Material and Methods

Patients

Between June 1982 and October 1997, 876 patients with esophageal cancer underwent esophagectomy with curative intent. All patients were subjected to detailed preoperative assessment of general status, organ function, and tumor stage according to the parameters listed in Table 1. All data from the preoperative assessment and the postoperative course were prospectively documented in a database.

The mode and extent of resection were standardized and determined by the location and histological type of the tumor as described elsewhere [7, 8]. A gastric tube was used for reconstruction in 777 patients and transverse/left hemicolon in 91. Esophagointestinal anastomosis was performed in the neck in 817 of 876 patients. Patients with cervical esophageal cancer and those who had resections with palliative intention were excluded from this study. The postoperative course was classified in each patient as defined in Table 2.

Table 1. Parameters used for preoperative assessment of patients with esophageal cancer

General Status	Sex
	Age
	Karnofsky Index [17] (0%–100%)
	History of alcohol abuse ("yes" or "no")
	History of tobacco abuse ("yes" or "no")
	Weight loss (in % of body weight)
	Mental cooperation of the patient ("good" or "poor")
Pulmonary function	Vital capacity (% of normal)
	Forced expiratory volume (FEV1, % of normal)
	Peak flow (% of normal)
	paO_2 (mmHg)
	$paCO_2$ (mmHg)
Hepatic function	Serum albumin (g/dl)
	Serum bilirubin (mg/dl)
	Partial thromboplastin time (sec)
	Aminopyrine breath test [14]
	Cirrhosis ("yes" or "no")
Renal function	Creatinine clearance (ml/min)
Cardiac function	ECG ("abnormal" or "normal")
	Chest x-ray ("abnormal" or "normal")
	Cardiologist's evaluation, with further detailed testing as indicated
	"normal risk", "increased risk", or "high risk"
Diabetes	"yes" or "no"

Tumor stage (based on standard staging techniques) [18, 19]: T1 or T2, locoregional; T3 or T4, locally advanced.

Table 2. Classification of postoperative course

Normal	Mechanical ventilation <48 h, ICU treatment 7 days
Prolonged	Mechanical ventilation 48 h–7 days or ICU treatment 7–21 days
Severe	Mechanical ventilation >7 days or ICU treatment >21 days, or readmission to ICU
Lethal	Death within 30 days

ICU, intensive care unit.

Study Design

The study was performed in three phases: In phase I, each of the preoperatively documented parameters was retrospectively correlated to the severity of postoperative course in 432 patients (377 men, 45 women, mean age 56.7 years) who had esophagectomy between June 1982 and December 1991. Discriminant analysis was performed to select the best cutoff point for parameters with an independent effect on multivariate analysis.

Based on the established parameters, preoperative organ function was classified as "normal", "compromised", or "severely impaired". The impact of individual organ dysfunction on postoperative mortality was subsequently assessed by regression analysis, and a composite score incorporating the risks of each individual organ system on postoperative mortality was established.

In phase II, the clinical value of the composite risk score predicting postoperative mortality was assessed in 121 patients (106 men, 15 women, mean age 57.9 years) who had esophagectomy for esophageal cancer between January 1992 and December 1993.

From January 1994 to October 1997 (phase III of the study), the composite risk score of each patient was included in the decision-making process for selection for surgical resection. During this period, 323 patients (265 men, 58 women, mean age 58.4 years) underwent esophagectomy. Patients at a high risk of preoperative death, based on the preoperative risk score, were referred to other modes of treatment. Nonsurgical treatment modalities were used in 31 patients with potentially resectable esophageal cancer but a high-risk score on preoperative analysis.

Statistical Analysis

All statistical analyses were performed with the BMDP statistical software package [9]. A p value below 0.05 was considered insignificant.

Results

Multivariate analysis showed a significant correlation between severity of postoperative course and preoperative Karnofsky index, the estimated mental "cooperation" of the patient, vital capacity, PaO_2 levels, the aminopyrine-breath-test (ABT), cirrhosis, and the presence of increased cardiac risk based on the cardiologist's judgement. The cutoff values which provide the best distinction between normal/prolonged and severe/lethal postoperative courses are shown in Table 3. Age, sex, tumor stage, the presence of diabetes, renal function, and history of alcohol or tobacco abuse had no independent effect on the postoperative course.

Based on the established parameters, each patient's hepatic, cardiac, and pulmonary functions and general status were individually classified as "nor-

Table 3. Cutoff values of individual independent continuous parameters providing the best distinction between normal/prolonged and severe/lethal postoperative course after esophagectomy (discriminant analysis in 432 patients undergoing esophagectomy between June 1982 and December 1991)

	Parameter	*p* Value
Karnofsky index	80%	<0.001
Aminopyrine breath test	0.4	<0.05
Vital capacity	90%	<0.05
paO_2	70 mmHg	<0.05

mal", "compromised", or "severely impaired" as shown in Table 4. Retrospective application of these scores to the 432 patients treated during phase I confirmed a significantly increased postoperative mortality for patients with severely impaired general status (relative risk 3.6), followed by poor cardiac function (relative risk 2.8), poor hepatic function (relative risk 2.1), and impaired respiratory function (relative risk 1.7).

In order to create a composite risk score for all relevant parameters, a weighing factor was established based on the relative risk associated with each individual factor. This factor was: general status × 4, cardiac function × 3, hepatic function × 2, and respiratory function × 2. Multiplying the individual preoperative cardiac, hepatic, and respiratory function and general status scores by this factor (Table 4) and adding the results creates a single composite score ranging from 11 points for a patient with no risk factors to 33 for patients with highest risk in all relevant parameters. Discriminant analysis showed that this composite scoring system enabled the patients to be divided into three distinct risk groups as regards postoperative mortality. Postoperative 30-day-mortality was 4.1% in the 194 patients with 11–15 points ("low-risk"), 9% in the 166 patients with 16–21 points ("moderate risk"), and 27.8% in the 72 patients with 22–33 points ("high-risk") ($p<0.05$ in all groups).

Prospective evaluation of this composite scoring system in 121 consecutive patients undergoing esophagectomy for esophageal cancer in phase II confirmed the validity of the scoring system in predicting postoperative course. Here, postoperative 30-day-mortality was 2.1% in the 46 patients classified as "low-risk" (11–15 points), 5.4% in the 55 patients classified as "moderate-risk" (16–21 points), and 25% in the 20 patients classified as "high-risk" (22–33 points) ($p<0.01$ for "low-risk" versus $p<0.05$ for "moderate risk").

The median score was 17 in 112 patients who survived the procedure, compared to a median score of 21 in the nine who died postoperatively ($p<0.01$). Of those nine, five were classified as "high-risk" on preoperative assessment, i.e., they had risk-scores of 22 or higher.

Including this composite scoring system into decision-making processes for selection for surgical resection and for excluding high-risk-patients from esophagectomy resulted in a marked decrease of postoperative mortality, down to 1.2% in our department after January 1994 (Table 5).

Table 4. Classification of individual organ dysfunction based on multivariate analysis of the postoperative course after esophagectomy

Pulmonary function	
Normal	VC>90% and paO_2>70 mmHg
Compromised	VC>90% or PAO_2<70 mmHg
Severely impaired	VC>90% and paO_2<70 mmHg
Hepatic function	
Normal	ABT>0.4
Compromised	ABT<0.4, no cirrhosis
Severely impaired	Cirrhosis
Cardiac function: based on cardiologist's impression	
Normal	Normal risk for major surgical procedure
Compromised	Increased risk for major surgical procedure
Severely impaired: high-risk patient for major surgical procedure	
General status	
Normal	Karnofsky index>80% and "good" co-operation
Compromised	Karnofsky index≤80% or "poor" co-operation
Severely impaired	Karnofsky index≤80% and "poor" cooperation

ABT, aminopyrine breath test; VC, vital capacity.

Table 5. Prevalence of "high risk" patients, i.e., patients with preoperative risk scores of 22 or higher and postoperative mortality from esophagectomy for esophageal cancer performed from 1982 to 1997 at the department of surgery, Munich Technical University

Time period	Total esophageal resections (*n*)	Prevalence of "high risk" patients	30-Day postoperative mortality
Phase I: June 1982–Dec 1991	432	72/432 (16.7%)	43/432 (9.9%)
Phase II: Jan 1992–Dec 1993	121	20/121 (16.5%)	9/121 (7.4%)
Phase III: Jan 1994–Oct 1997	323	27/323 (8.4%)	4/323 (1.2%)

Discussion

Surgeons' experience and training and physiological status of patients have been clearly identified as main risk factors affecting mortality of esophagectomy for esophageal cancer [2, 3, 6, 10]. Postoperative mortality in experienced centers can be reduced further only by better recognition of patients with sufficient physiological reserves to withstand the extended surgical procedure and potentially complicated postoperative course. The present study shows that the risk of postoperative death in patients with resectable esophageal cancer is determined, in decreasing order, by preoperative general status and cardiac, hepatic, and respiratory functions. Objective assessment of preoperative function of these organ systems and calculation of a composite score based on the relative impact of each individual parameter allowed us to establish "low-", "moderate-", and "high-" risk groups for esophageal resection. This score provides an objective instrument in the patient selection process.

General status has been difficult to categorize objectively [2, 4, 6, 11]. Judgment of the patient's mental cooperation by a surgeon is undoubtely subjective and introduces a nonquantifiable aspect into the proposed score. Attributes of "poor" or "good" cooperation alone, without taking into account other, objective parameters, did not cause marked changes in composite scores.

Pulmonary and cardiac complications account for up to 70% of postoperative deaths after esophagectomy [2, 4, 11–13]. This is reflected in the rather high factor attributed to cardiac dysfunction. Detailed cardiological evaluation is therefore recommended in any patient being considered for esophagectomy whose history, physical examination, EKG, or chest x-rays show any abnormality. Spirometric parameters have not consistently been found useful in predicting pulmonary complications after major surgery [11, 13]. This and other analyses [2, 15] show that measuring vital capacity in combination with PaO_2 allows identification of patients with increased risk of postoperative death after esophagectomy. Routine preoperative pulmonary function tests are therefore recommended before considering esophagectomy.

Decompensated liver cirrhosis is considered a contraindication for esophageal resection in many centers. An independent effect of hepatic dysfunction on postoperative mortality rate is confirmed also by the present study. It shows that the aminopyrine breath test, which assesses hepatic cytochrome p450 function, allows identification of patients at increased risk of postoperative mortality, even in the absence of cirrhosis [14]. This noninvasive and easy test should therefore be included in assessment of hepatic function in any patient being considered for esophageal resection.

In contrast to other reports [2, 3] tumor stage and patient age did not predict postoperative death in the present analysis. This is most likely due to the extensive preoperative tumor staging performed at our institution, which usually allows identification and exlusion of patients with metastatic or irresectable tumours before operation. Our study further shows that advanced age alone is not associated with increased risk of postoperative death. Similar to the experience reported by Peracchia et al. [16], ours indicates that the benefits of a potentially curative resection should not be withheld from otherwise fit patients with resectable tumors simply because of advanced age.

In summary, the present study shows that the risk of esophagectomy in patients with potentially resectable esophageal cancer can be assessed objectively before operation and quantified by a composite risk score. Consistently including the risk score in the preoperative decision-making process resulted in a marked decrease of postoperative mortality to less than 2% at our institution. This risk score may therefore be used to refine the criteria for selection or choice of procedure in patients for esophageal resection.

References

1. Müller JM, Erasmi H, Stelzner M, Zieren U, Pichlmaier H (1990) Surgical therapy of esophageal carcinoma. Br J Surg 77:845–855
2. Law SYK, Fok M, Wong J (1994) Risk analysis in resection of squamous cell carcinoma of the oesophagus. World J Surg 18:339–346
3. Lund O, Kimose HH, Aagaard MT, Hasenkam JM, Erlandsen M (1990) Risk stratification and long-term results after surgical treatment of carcinomas of the thoracic oesophagus and cardia. J Thorac Cardiovasc Surg 99:200–209
4. Bartels H, Stein HJ, Schömig A, Siewert JR (1997) Risikoerfassung. Chirurg 68:654–661
5. Bartels H, Stein HJ, Siewert JR (1998) Preoperative risk analysis and postoperative mortality of oesophagectomy for resectable esophageal cancer. Br J Surg (in press)
6. Bumm R, Panel of experts (1996) Staging and risk analysis in esophageal carcinoma. Results of a consensus conference. Dis Esoph 9 [Suppl]:20–29
7. Siewert JR, Bartels H, Bollschweiler E et al (1992) Plattenepithelcarcinom des Oesophagus. Behandlungskonzept der Chirurgischen Klinik der Technischen Universität München. Chirurg 63:693–700
8. Siewert JR, Hölscher AH, Bollschweiler E, Stein HJ, Fink U (1994) Chirurgie des Barrett-Carcinoms. Chirurg 66:102–109
9. Dixon WJ (1988) BMDP statistical software manual. University of California Press, Berkeley CA
10. Mathews HR, Powell DJ, McCarley CL (1986) Effect of surgical experience on results of resection for oesophageal carcinoma. Br J Surg 63:621–633
11. Tsutsui S, Moriguchi S, Moritha M, Kuwano H, Matsuda H, Mori M, Matsuura H, Sugimachi K (1992) Multivariate analysis of postoperative complications after oesophageal resection. Ann N Thorac Surg 53:1052–1056
12. Isono K, Onoda S, Ishikawa T, Sato H, Nahayama K (1982) Studies on the causes of deaths from oesophageal carcinoma. Cancer 49:2173–2179
13. Nishi M, Hiramatsu J, Hioki K, Hatano T, Yamamota M (1988) Pulmonary complications after subtotal oesophagectomy. Br J Surg 75:527–530
14. Gill R, Goodman N, Golfus G (1983) Aminopyrine breath test predicts surgical risk for patients with liver disease. Ann Surg 198:701–704
15. Fun S, Lau WY, Yip WC et al (1987) Prediction of postoperative pulmonary complications in oesophagogastric cancer surgery. Br J Surg 74:408–410
16. Peracchia A, Bardini R, Ruol A et al (1988) Carcinoma of the oesophagus in the elderly: indications and results of surgery. Dis Esoph 1:147–153
17. Karnofsky D (1984) Reporting results of cancer treatment. Cancer 1:634–635
18. Siewert JR, Dittler H-J (1993) Oesophageal carcinoma: impact of staging on treatment. Endoscopy 25:28–32
19. Dittler H-J, Siewert JR (1993) Role of endoscopic ultrasonography in esophageal cancer. Endoscopy 25:156–161

Neoadjuvant Chemoradiation Followed by Surgery for Resectable Esophageal Cancer

R. F. Heitmiller, A. A. Forastiere, L. Kleinberg, M. Zahurak

Departments of Surgery and Oncology at The Johns Hopkins Medical Institutions, Baltimore, Maryland, USA

Abstract

Neoadjuvant chemoradiation (NAC) therapy protocols were developed to improve survival in patients with resectable esophageal cancer. Our experience with two consecutive NAC therapy trials is reviewed. Both studies included patients with localized squamous cell cancer and adenocarcinoma. Patients were treated with cisplatinum 26 mg/m^2/day (days 1–5 and 26–30), 5-Flourouracil (5-FU) 300 mg/m^2/day (days 1–30), concurrent radiotherapy (4400 cGy) followed by esophagectomy. In the second trial, adjuvant taxol was added. The first protocol had 50 patients. Two patients died, both before surgery, one from sepsis. There was no residual viable tumor (CR) in 19 (40%) patients. The median survial time was 31 months. The 5-year survival rate of 36% compared favorably with concurrent 5-year survival of 18% for surgery alone. Fourty-one patients were enrolled in the second trial. All underwent surgery. There were no treatment or operative deaths. Survival data for this group is maturing. Combined results from both protocols are: treatment mortality of 2.2%, complete response rate of 37%, and a median and 3-year disease-specific survival of 42 months and 54%, respectively. We conclude that NAC followed by surgery improves survival over surgery alone and that CR is predictive of improved survival.

Introduction

Postesophagectomy survival is stage-related, with survival falling sharply with increasing stage. Recent advances in esophagectomy technique and perioperative management which has significantly reduced surgical morbidity, mortality, and length of hospital stay have not been associated with improved postresection survival. The majority of esophageal cancer patients present with locally advanced staged, or AJCC stages 2 and 3 tumors. For these patients, postresection survival remains limited. NAC therapy protocols were developed in order to improve survival in patients with resectable esophageal cancer. Our experience with NAC therapy at The Johns Hopkins Hospital is reviewed.

Recent Results in Cancer Research, Vol. 155

Initial Trial

Investigators at the University of Michigan reported that 3 weeks of preoperative cisplatinum, 5-FU, and Velban with concurrent radiotherapy followed by esophagectomy resulted in a 24% complete histologic response rate and a 5-year survival rate of 35% [1]. We modified this treatment plan by deleting Velban and increasing the treatment interval to 4 weeks in order to reduce toxicity and permit outpatient therapy [2].

Patients and Methods

The study was open to patients with squamous cell carcinoma or adenocarcinoma of the esophagus or gastroesophageal junction whose disease was localized and could be encompassed in a single radiation port. Patients with locoregional adenopathy were eligible for treatment. Patients had to be surgical candidates, both in terms of resectability and acceptable surgical risks, prior to neoadjuvant therapy. Other eligibility criteria included a Karnofsky scale performance status of 60% or greater, adequate bone marrow reserve (WBC and platelet count equal to or greater than 3500 and 100,000 cells/μl, respectively), and adequate renal function (creatinine clearance equal to or greater than 50 cc/min).

The treatment plan is summarized in Fig. 1. Patients were treated with cisplatinum 26 mg/m^2/day continuous infusion on days 1–5 and 26–30. 5-FU 300 mg/m^2/day was administered as a continuous infusion on days 1–30, throughout the entire course of radiotherapy. Radiation was administered using a four-field technique (AP, PA, and two lateral ports) with the patient in the prone position. Daily fractions of 200 cGy, 5 days per week were delivered, to a total dose of 4400 cGy. The neoadjuvant therapy was followed by a 4-week recovery period, with surgery targeted for day 58. Minimum requirements for surgery were a white blood cell count of 3000 cells/μl, platelet count of 100,000 cells/μl, and clinical assessment of recovery. Esophagectomy technique varied according to the patient, the level of disease, and the individual surgeon. The transhiatal approach was favored, reflecting the first author's preference and the high proportion of adenocarcinomas. Patients

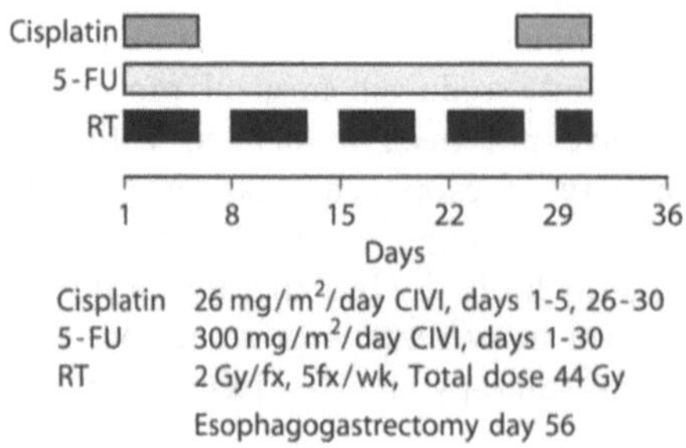

Fig. 1. The first neoadjuvant chemoradiation therapy followed by surgery protocol is summarized. *Cisplat*, cisplatinum; *5-FU*, 5-flourouracil; *RT*, radiotherapy

were managed postoperatively as previously reported [3]. The pathology was reviewed and tumors staged using the AJCC tumor node metastasis (TNM) classification [4].

Results

Fifty patients were entered into this protocol with a mean age of 60 (range: 32–74) years. There were 33 patients with adenocarcinoma (66%), 16 with squamous cell cancer (32%), and one with undifferentiated carcinoma (2%). Patient demographics reflected the high proportion of adenocarcinoma, with 42 males, eight females, 46 white, and four African-American patients. No attempt was made to select patients with early-staged tumors. Pretreatment staging by contrast esophagogram and computed tomography demonstrated tumor length >5 cm in 39 (78%), circumferential or obstructing tumors in 19 (38%), and enlarged lymph nodes in 18 (36%).

Results of the chemoradiation therapy are summarized in Table 1. Two patients died prior to surgery, one from leukopenia and sepsis. One patient was found to have miliary abdominal metastatic disease and was classified as a patient with progression of disease on therapy. Grade 3 or 4 leukopenia was documented in 40 (80%) and nausea and vomiting in 41 (80%) patients. Weight loss was <5% in 33 (66%) patients; however, intravenous total nutritional support (TPN) was used in 25 (50%) patients.

A total of 47 patients underwent surgical resection for an operability rate of 94%. The operative technique used was transhiatal in 35, three-incision approach in nine, and left thoracoabdominal in three patients (Table 2). The operative procedure was thought potentially curative in 45 of 47 (90%) patients. Surgical results are summarized in Table 3. No patients died from surgery, regardless of length of hospital stay. The mean length of stay in intensive care and hospital overall was 2.1 and 15 days, respectively. The compli-

Table 1. Results of chemoradiation therapy

	Number of patients (%)
Mortality	2 (4%)
Disease progression	1 (2%)
Grade 3 or 4 leukopenia	40 (80%)
Nausea or vomiting	41 (80%)
Weight loss >5%	13 (26%)
TPN	25 (50%)

Table 2. Surgical technique

Transhiatal 35 (29 ADENO, 6 SCCA)
Three-incision approach 9 (9 SCCA)
Left thoracoabdominal 3 (3 ADENO)

Table 3. Results of surgical therapy

Result	Number of patients (%)
Mortality	0 (0%)
Overall morbidity	17 (36%)
Anastomotic leak	1 (2%)
Abdominal wound infection	1 (2%)
Pneumonia	0 (0%)

Table 4. Pathology results

AJCC Stage	Number of patients (%)
Pathologic CR	19 (40%)
1	5 (11%)
2A	10 (21%)
2B	7 (15%)
3	5 (11%)
4	1 (2%)

cation rate was 36%. Most of these were minor and did not affect the duration of hospital stay. Despite the high incidence of chemoradiation-induced leukopenia, there were few infectious complications. One patient (2%) had a cervical anastomotic leak which was treated by cervical drainage with subsequent closure, and one patient (2%) developed an abdominal wound infection which was succesfully treated by incision, drainage, and dressings. No patient developed pneumonia.

Postresection pathology is summarized in Table 4. There was no residual viable tumor (pathologic complete response) in 19 (40%) patients. A total of 22 patients (47%) were either stage 2 or 3, five patients (11%) had stage 1, and one patient (2%) had stage 4 disease.

Overall survival for the entire group, including treatment-related deaths, is shown in Fig. 2. The median survival time was 31 months and the 5-year survival rate was 36%. Historical controls have reported notably consistent postesophagectomy 5-year survival rates of 20%–22% [5–7]. We reviewed our postesophagectomy 5-year survival results in patients managed without neoadjuvant chemoradiation therapy. Although not a prospective randomized comparison, this series was performed by the same surgeon at the same institution and concurrent with our NAC protocol. We showed an overall post-esophagectomy survival rate of 18%. The overall survival rates between adenocarcinoma and squamous cell cancers were the same [8]. Although there was a trend towards longer median survival in patients with adenocarcinoma, there was no difference in overall 5-year survival by cell type. Another recent review of postsurgical survival with NAC therapy revealed similar findings, with an overall 5-year survival level of 25%. Therefore, our results

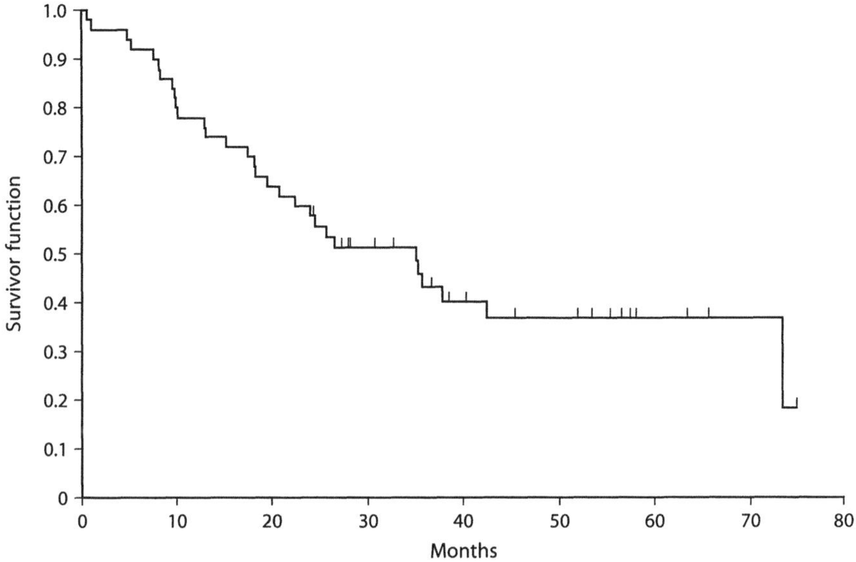

Fig. 2. Kaplan-Meier survival curve for the 50 patients in the first protocol. (From [2])

suggested a survival benefit in patients treated with NAC therapy. Furthermore, when survival rate was between those with pathologic complete response (CR) and those with residual viable tumor, regardless of stage, were compared, a significant survival advantage was demonstrated for the CR patients as illustrated in Fig. 3. Of the 20 patients with tumor recurrence, 19 (95%) presented with distant metastatic disease only, and one (5%) presented with local and distal disease.

Second Trial

Based on our experience with NAC in the first 50 patients, a second neoadjuvant chemoradiation therapy protocol was opened. The NAC was identical to that used in the first protocol. Patients were staged with chest and abdominal computed tomography, endoscopic ultasound, and laparoscopy in order to determine preoperative TNM staging as accurately as possible. Improved pretherapy staging would ensure appropriate patient selection and permit documentation of the apparent "downstaging" seen in the first protocol. Recurrent disease following the first NAC protocol was outside of the radiation and surgical fields in the form of distant, metastatic disease. Therefore, in the second protocol, postoperative adjuvant taxol was added to enhance systemic control of tumor and to improve survival.

In total, 41 patients have been entered onto the second protocol, which is now closed. There were no deaths from either chemoradiation therapy or

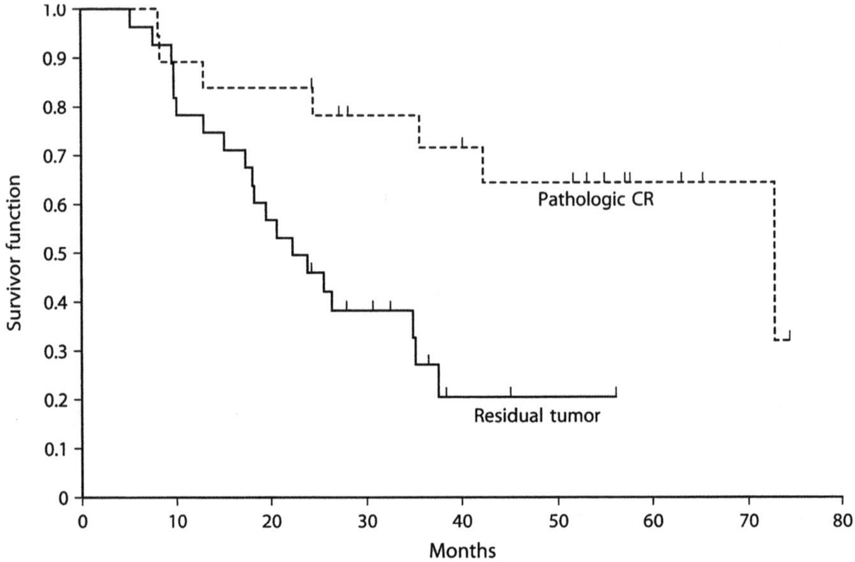

Fig. 3. Kaplan-Meier survival curve based on pathologic response. *Pathologic CR*, complete response (no residual viable tumor). (From [2])

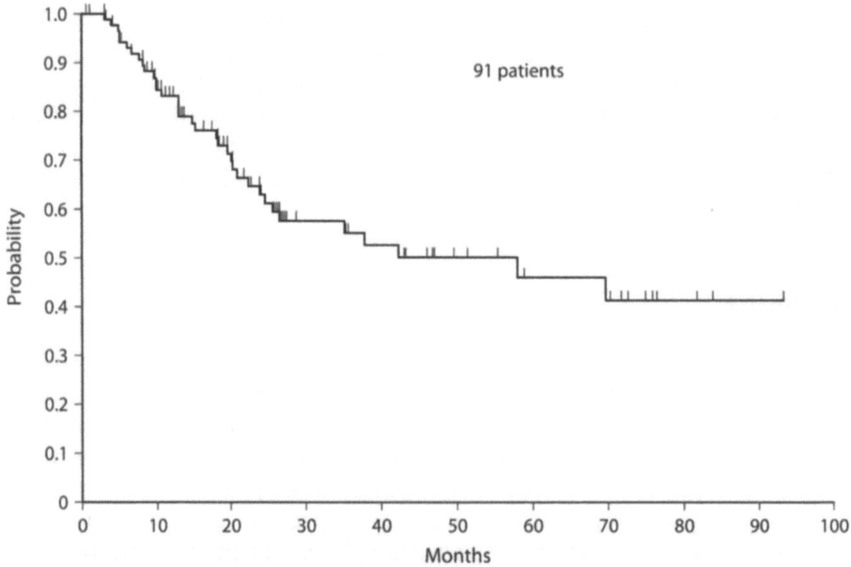

Fig. 4. Kaplan-Meier survival curve for 91 patients, combined from both protocols

subsequent surgery. Survival data for this group is maturing. Combining both protocols for a total of 91 patients, the following results are obtained [9]: pathologic complete response was seen in 37% (Fig. 4), and the median and 3-year disease-specific Kaplan-Meier overall survival times were 42 months and 54%, respectively. Patients with a pathologic complete response continue to show a significant survival advantage, as shown in Fig. 5. When survival data is evaluated by cell type, no significance difference is demonstrated (Fig. 6).

Conclusions

Based on our experience with NAC for resectable esophageal carcinoma, we conclude that NAC followed by surgery does appear to improve survival over surgery alone. The therapy is associated with acceptable toxicity, morbidity, and mortality. Complete pathologic response to preoperative chemoradiation therapy is predictive of improved survival. Overall post-treatment survival does not appear to be affected by cell type.

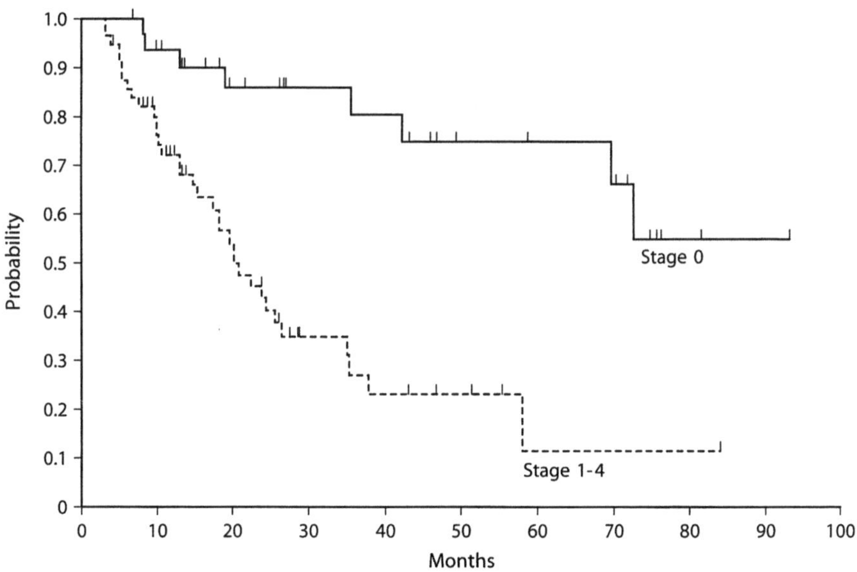

Fig. 5. Kaplan-Meier survival curves for 91 patients by pathologic stage. Stage 0 patients denote no residual viable disease

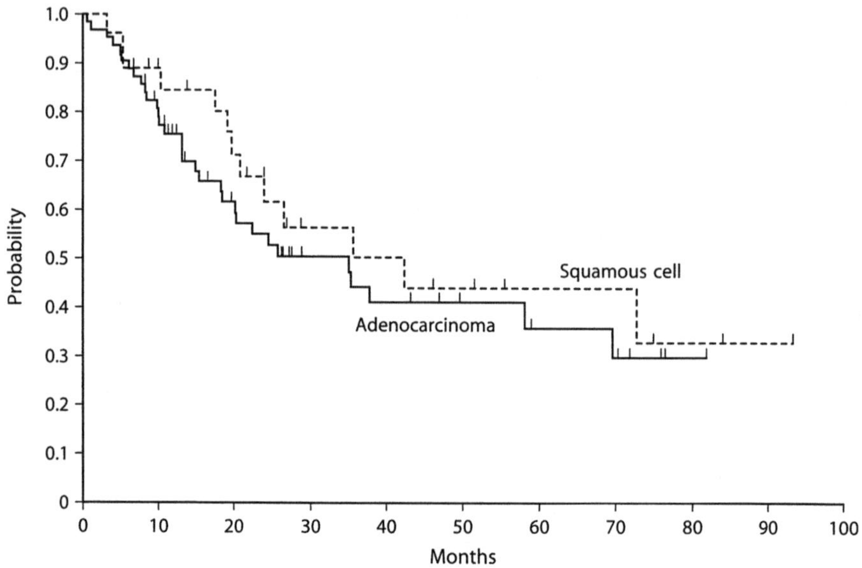

Fig. 6. Kaplan-Meier survival curves for 91 patients by cell type

References

1. Forastiere AA, Orringer MB, Perez-Tamayo C et al (1993) Preoperative chemoradiation followed by transhiatal esophagectomy for carcinoma of the esophagus: final report. J Clin Oncol 6:1118–1123
2. Forastiere AA, Heitmiller RF, Lee D-J, Zahurak M, Abrams R, Kleinberg L, Watkins S, Yeo CJ, Lillemoe KD, Sitzman JV, Sharfman W (1997) Intensive chemoradiation therapy followed by esophagectomy for squamous cell and adenocarcinoma of the esophagus. Cancer J Sci Am 3:144–52
3. Gillinov AM, Heitmiller RF (1998) Strategies to reduce pulmonary complications after transhiatal esophagectomy. Dis Esophag 11:43–47
4. American Joint Committee on Cancer (1988) Manual for staging of cancer, 3rd edn. Lippincott, Philadelphia
5. Ellis FH Jr (1989) Treatment of carcinoma of the esophagus and gastric cardia. Mayo Clin Proc 64:945–955
6. King MR, Pairolero PC, Trastek VF, Payne WS, Bernatz PE (1987) Ivor-Lewis esophagogastrectomy for carcinoma of the esophagus: early and late functional results. Ann Thorac Surg 44:119–22
7. Wilkins EW Jr, Wong J (eds) (1988) Mosby, St Louis, pp 440–444
8. Salazar JD, Doty JR, Lin JW, Dyke MC, Roberts J, Heitmiller ES, Heitmiller RF (1998) Does cell type influence postesophagectomy survival in patients with esophageal cancer? Dis Esophag 11:168–71
9. Ellis FH Jr, Heatley GJ, Krasna MJ, Williamson WA, Balogh K (1997) Esophagogastrectomy for carcinoma of the esophagus and cardia: a comparison of findings and results after standard resection in three consecutive eight-year intervals with improved staging criteria. J Thorac Cardiovasc Surg 113:836–846

Neoadjuvant Therapy of Squamous Cell Carcinoma of the Esophagus

D. P. Kelsen

Memorial Sloan Kettering Cancer Center, Department of Medicine,
Gastrointestinal Oncology Service, 1275 York Avenue, New York, NY 10021, USA

Abstract

Because of the high risk of recurrence following surgery for squamous cell carcinomas of the esophagus, treatment involving both systemic therapy and a localized approach [either surgery alone or chemo/radiation and surgery] have been extensively studied. Pilot trials have demonstrated safety for the use of chemotherapy followed by operation, or for chemotherapy plus standard radiation plus surgery. Larger scale phase III trials, in which either of these two strategies is employed, have now been reported. For chemotherapy followed by surgery, conflicting results have recently been noted. A US intergroup trial showed no significant outcome for all patients treated. A smaller European study, also using a cisplatin-based regimen, had a positive result. Similarly, for chemoradiation followed by operation, two recent random assignment studies falled to demonstrate a significant difference in outcome. However, recently newer chemotherapy agents have been identified which hold promise for more effective therapy. These include paclitaxel and irinotecan. Phase II trials, using these agents prior to surgery, are underway or have been completed, and phase III studies are in the advanced planning stage. Until these trials have demonstrated superiority, surgery alone or chemoradiation without surgery remain the standard of care, for patients with esophageal cancer.

Introduction

Esophageal carcinoma, a virulent malignancy with an overall poor prognosis, has become more common in the United States over the last 15 years. While the incidence of epidermoid carcinomas of the esophagus has remained relatively constant, adenocarcinoma has become increasingly more common [1]. At the present time, the general approach to both histologic subtypes is similar.

For patients with tumors limited to the local regional area (T1–3NanyM0), there are two potentially curative therapies available. The first is surgical resection, and the second is the combination of chemotherapy and concurrent radiation. A combined approach involving systemic chemotherapy and at least one local modality is an attractive concept because of the high distant failure rate and significant local recurrence risk when surgery or radiation alone are used. In addition, a subgroup of patients present with such extensive local regional tumor (T4) that resection is impossible and results with radiation alone are unsatisfactory. In this situation, chemotherapy prior to surgery or concurrently with radiation is used in a group of patients who do not, as currently staged, have curable disease. This paper will focus on recent neoadjuvant studies in patients with epidermoid carcinoma of the esophagus.

Failure Pattern

As is the case with many solid tumors, knowing the potential failure pattern after curative intent treatment is crucial in order to best plan new therapies. Tumors that have a high local failure rate, but infrequently metastasize to distant sites (e.g., low-grade sarcomas), might best be treated by use of aggressive surgery with or without radiation therapy (either external beam or brachytherapy). In this situation, systemic therapy is used primarily as a radiation sensitizer. On the other hand, for a tumor with a high risk for systemic metastasis with or without a high local failure rate, the use of systemic therapy early in the treatment plan is quite rational. This is why neoadjuvant chemotherapy (also known as preoperative or primary chemotherapy) is a particularly attractive concept for several solid tumors [2]. For esophageal cancer, the major data available for failure pattern after potentially curative local regional therapy come from clinical reviews and from autopsy series. There is no substantial body of information from planned second-look operations. The data from autopsy series and selected clinical trials have been previously reported. In brief, distant failure is a common event in both autopsy and clinical reviews, with liver, lung, and lymph nodes being the most common site of recurrence. Local failure occurs clinically in up to one third of patients both in autopsy series and in clinical studies.

Theoretical Rationale for Chemotherapy Plus Radiation

Volkes and others have reviewed the rationale for the combination of chemotherapy given concurrently with radiation [2]. The two modalities may have independent activity against different tumor cell subpopulations. Cells that are intrinsically resistant to one modality may be sensitive to the other. This remains to be proven on a clinical basis, since this hypothesis is controversial; laboratory experiments show that a mutated p53 gene, for example, confers relative resistance both to chemotherapy and radiation. The use of combined modality therapy might allow destruction of resistant cell populations, preventing later cellular expansion of subgroups of tumor cells. Chemotherapy may delay the regrowth of tumor cell populations that were sensitive to radiation, and this delay in regrowth may increase total cell kill when the next radiation dose is given. By causing cell cycle synchronization or blocking cancer cells in the phase most sensitive to radiation (G_2M), chemotherapy may be synergistic with radiation. Lastly, chemoradiation interactions might improve as the tumor grows smaller, since oxygenation in the center portions of a smaller mass may be better, leading to improved radiation cell kill. In a second review, Steel and Peckem proposed three additional mechanisms of enhanced chemoradiation interaction [3]. Spatial cooperation means that radiation will have a high degree of locoregional activity, while chemotherapy is active both locally and systemically. Spatial cooperation, however, does not necessarily require the two modalities to begiven concurrently. Independent toxicity profiles may allow full doses of both modalities to be used, although in fact substantial clinical data suggest that, for many drugs, the dose of chemotherapy given must be attenuated when concurrent radiation is employed. Finally, the development of radiation sensitizers that increase the therapeutic index of radiation by giving normal tumor protection is a theoretical goal which has not yet been completely achieved. Alternatively, technical improvements in radiation (such as confrontational planning) may allow higher total doses of radiation to the tumor while better protecting local structures.

Choice of the Appropriate Patient for Adjuvant Therapy

High-risk esophageal cancer patients are those who have tumors that are still potentially curable but have stages T3 or T4, or have lymph node metastasis, but have no evidence of distant disease (stages IIA–IIB, III). Definitive staging is usually assigned postoperatively after resection of the primary esophageal tumor. Survival outcome by stage has been reported by many authors. Even patients with T3N0 tumors have a greater than 50% chance of recurrence and death within 5 years of resection, while those with lymph node metastasis have an even more ominous prognosis. A total of 80%–90% of Western patients fall in the high-risk group. Preoperative staging to identify patients at lower risk is still in the developmental stage; however, recent studies indicate that two new techniques may be superior to traditional use of barium esophagram, computed tomography (CT) scanning, or magnetic resonance imaging (MRI) of the chest and abdomen. Neither CT nor MRI are accurate in staging T or regional lymph node involvement. Endoscopic ultrasonography (EUS) has been shown to be highly accurate for assessing depth of penetration and may improve staging of nodal disease as well [4, 5]. For tumors at the esophagogastric junction, laparoscopy as a staging tool, sometimes with the use of laparoscopy ultrasonography, has demonstrated the ability to identify small-volume peritoneal metastasis or small-volume hepatic metastasis. Lastly, positron emission tomography (PET) scanning is now in extensive clinical trial and shows promise for better assessment of nodal and other distant metastasis.

Once the patient has been identified as being at high risk for recurrence, the question of adjuvant or neoadjuvant therapy is appropriately asked.

Postoperative Chemotherapy

For several common solid tumors, such as breast or colon cancers, postoperative adjuvant therapy has been widely employed. Large-scale random assignment trials have clearly demonstrated a statistically and clinically significant decrease in recurrence following definitive locoregional therapy, which has translated to an absolute increase in the cure rate. However, for esophageal cancer, postoperative adjuvant therapy, either consisting of radiation following resection or of chemotherapy following resection, has not been demonstrated to increase cure rates. This may be because of an inability to deliver effective doses of active chemotherapeutic agents in this population following major chest and abdominal surgery, because chemotherapeutic agents currently employed are simply not effective enough, or because the delay in starting postoperative treatment increases the likelihood that subclinical metastases will grow to the point of incurability. The major interest in the last 10–15 years has therefore been in the neoadjuvant approach.

Neoadjuvant Therapy

The three major approaches for combined modality therapy that have been explored in patients with localized esophageal cancers are preoperative chemotherapy alone followed by an operation, chemoradiation followed by operation, or chemotherapy and radiation without operation. After phase II trials demonstrated the safety of all these techniques, random assignment studies were performed. The remainder of this chapter will summarize random assignment studies.

Chemotherapy Followed by Operation

Several small, random assignment trials were performed in the early to mid-1980s and have been previously summarized in detail [6]. These studies all demonstrated that preoperative chemotherapy involving cisplatin-containing combinations was well tolerated, without any increase in operative morbidity or mortality. Response rates, when measured by barium esophagram, varied widely, ranging from 25% to 50%. No definitive conclusions regarding an improvement in survival could be drawn from these earlier studies, either because of their relatively small size, which significantly limited the power of the trial, or because of a crossover design which allowed surgery patients to receive chemotherapy postoperatively [7–9].

More recently, two large-scale studies have been reported in which patients with either epidermoid carcinoma alone or epidermoid and adenocarcinoma patients were randomly assigned to surgery alone or to preoperative chemotherapy followed by operation. No crossover was allowed in these trials. Kok et al. reported in abstract form the final results of a random assignment trial comparing preoperative cisplatin and etoposide chemotherapy followed by operation to operation alone. This study, which was performed in the Netherlands, involved the use of up to four cycles of cisplatin (80 mg/m^2) per day and etoposide (100 mg IV days 1 and 2 followed by 200 mg/m^2 oral doses on days 3 and 5). Surgery consisted of a transhiatal esophagectomy with a gastric anastomosis. During the period 1990–1996, 160 patients were treated; 148 were evaluable for analysis. Chemotherapy was reasonably well tolerated, although there was one treatment-related death due to neutropenic sepsis. An overall major objective response rate to chemotherapy of 36% was reported. The resection rates were similar between the two groups. With a median follow-up of 15 months, the median survival for patients receiving preoperative chemotherapy was 18.5 months versus 11 months for patients undergoing operation alone (p=0.002). The authors concluded that neoadjuvant chemotherapy prolongs survival in patients with operable tumors.

In a second, larger study, also available in preliminary abstract form, Kelsen and colleagues reported the preliminary results of a USA National Intergroup trial (Intergroup 113). This study involved patients both with adenocarcinoma and epidermoid cancer. A total of 444 patients were evaluable, of which 205 had epidermoid carcinoma. The study involved randomization between operation alone versus up to three cycles of cisplatin–fluorouracil chemotherapy followed by operation. Patients in the neoadjuvant group who underwent a potentially curative (R0) resection were to have received two additional postoperative cycles of the same chemotherapy at a lower dose of cisplatin. Transhiatal esophagectomy was allowed in this study only for tumors in the distal third of the esophagus, with most patients having a procedure involving thoracotomy.

Chemotherapy was also well tolerated in this study, with a 2% treatment-related mortality. There was no increase in operative morbidity or mortality comparing the neoadjuvant chemotherapy group to patients undergoing surgery alone. In this large-scale national trial, the operative mortality rate for patients receiving surgery alone was 6%, while the rate for patients receiving chemotherapy prior to surgery was 5% (not significant). However, while chemotherapy was well tolerated and did not increase operative complications, there was no significant increase in survival. In addition, there was no significant difference in survival for either histologic subgroup in an overall comparison. In other words, patients with epidermoid cancer had the same survival outcome with or without chemotherapy as did patients with adenocarcinoma.

The conflicting results of these two studies may be a result of a difference in effectiveness in the chemotherapy regimen (although this has not been shown in patients with more advanced disease) or may be a function of the size of the trials. Further, the median duration of survival in patients undergoing operation alone in the larger U.S. trial was 16.2 months, while in the trial from the Netherlands the median survival was only 11.5 months.

The differing results of these two studies indicate that the use of chemotherapy followed by operation remains an investigational approach. Newer, more effective forms of systemic chemotherapy have been identified, which are now entering combined modality studies. These include paclitaxel and irinotecan base combinations. These studies are still in phase I and II of development.

Chemoradiation Followed by Operation

As is the case for chemotherapy followed by surgery, chemoradiation followed by surgery has also undergone extensive phase II trials demonstrating general tolerance to this approach. Earlier studies involved relatively small numbers of patients, and no definitive conclusions could be reached. More recently, four trials have been performed involving the technique of chemoradiation followed by operation. Two of these involve patients with adenocarcinoma, and two have been limited to patients with epidermoid carcinoma. While the studies by Walsh et al. and in preliminary abstract form by Urba et al. indicated an advantage to chemoradiation followed by transhiatal esophagectomy, an opposite result was found in larger-scale studies in epidermoid cancer.

LePrise and colleagues treated a total of 86 patients with localized squamous cell carcinoma of the esophagus using a technique of chemotherapy followed by radiation and then operation. In this trial, it is important to note that chemotherapy was not given concurrently with radiation, i.e., cisplatin and fluorouracil were given from days 1–5 on cycle 1; radiation was given on day 8 and completed on day 19 (total dose 20 cGy in ten fractions over 12 days). A second cycle of chemotherapy was given beginning on day 21. Surgery was scheduled to be performed on day 42. In addition, this study was initially planned to have 150 patients and did not have a planned interim analysis. While chemoradiation therapy was reasonably well tolerated and did not increase operative morbidity or mortality, there was no significant difference in survival; at 3 years, 19.2% of chemoradiation patients were alive versus 13.8% of patients receiving surgery only.

In a larger, more recent study, Bosset et al. compared cisplatin radiation therapy followed by operation versus operation alone, also in patients with epidermoid cancer of the esophagus. The total dose of radiation was 37 Gy given in ten 3.7-Gy fractions. Thus chemoradiation therapy was sequential rather than concurrent. A total of 282 patients were evaluable, 139 receiving surgery alone and 143 receiving chemoradiation followed by operation. Although chemotherapy and radiation were reasonably well tolerated, there was a significant increase in operative mortality for patients receiving preoperative chemotherapy compared with those undergoing operation alone (17 of 138 vs. 5 of 137, $p=0.012$). The curative resection rate was higher in patients receiving combined chemoradiation than in those undergoing operation alone (p=0.017). There was no significant difference in overall survival for the two groups of patients. With a median follow-up of 55.2 months, the median survival was 18.6 months for both arms. Cancer deaths were, however, more common in the group receiving surgery alone, and the authors concluded that the high operative mortality may have had a impact on the lack of benefit seen for chemoradiation therapy patients.

The contrasting results of these two sets of trials in epidermoid and in adenocarcinoma patients make the use of chemoradiation therapy followed by operation also still an investigational approach. A large scale USA Intergroup trial has just been initiated which should definitively test the hypothesis that cisplatin-fluorouracil plus concurrent radiation followed by operation is a superior treatment in terms of overall survival when compared to surgery alone.

Chemoradiation Without Operation

Several trials designed in the mid- to late 1980s have tested the hypothesis that chemoradiation therapy is superior to radiation alone in patients with esophageal cancer. The majority of patients in these early studies had epidermoid carcinoma. In the best-known trial, reported on behalf of the RTOG and Southwestern Oncology Group (SWOG) by Herskovitz and colleagues, a total of 121 patients were randomly assigned to receive either a higher-dose radiation therapy (6400 cGy) or radiation (5000 cGy) plus concurrent cisplatin-fluorouracil. The trial, which was originally planned to have 2409 patients in total, was stopped at an interim analysis when a statically significant survival advantage was shown for the patients receiving chemoradiation therapy.

The contrasting results of the RTOG 85-01 trial using an almost identical chemotherapy as that employed in the Intergroup 113 trial (cisplatin plus fluorouracil) are also somewhat confusing. It is not clear whether chemoradiation therapy without operation is superior to chemotherapy followed by operation or whether the small number of patients in the RTOG 85-01 trial found a survival advantage that may not be maintained in large groups of patients. Larger-scale confirmatory trials are currently underway in the United States in which patients with both adenocarcinoma and epidermoid cancer are randomly assigned to either receive treatment identical to that of the experimental arm of the RTOG 85-01 trial (cisplatin-fluorouracil plus 5000 cGy of radiation) or to a higher dose of radiation (6400 cGy plus the same agents). Almost 200 patients have been registered for this study to date. The results of the trial will be available in approximately 2 years.

Future Directions

The ability to safely give chemotherapy prior to operation with or without radiation or, in a nonoperative approach, concurrently with radiation has been demonstrated. Encouraging results suggest a survival advantage in nonoperative therapy of combined concurrent radiation and chemotherapy. Clearly, however, better systemic agents are need. Two new agents with activity in esophageal cancer have recently been identified: paclitaxel and the camptothecan irinotecan. Phase I and phase II trials using the technique of chemotherapy and concurrent radiation alone or chemotherapy and radiation followed by operation using paclitaxel-containing regimens are being tested at a number of centers, with large-scale random assignment trials planned for the future. These newer agents, which appear to have more activity than cisplatin–fluorouracil, hold promise for improving the distant failure rate, which remains a major problem in increasing the cure rate in patients with esophageal cancer. Furthermore, molecular markers obtained from tumor biopsies, such as thymidylate synthase, dipyrimidine dehydrogenase, thymidine phosphorylase, excision repair gene (ERCC-1) and tubulin isoforms, show promise for allowing individualization of chemotherapy regimens on the basis of pretreatment tumor characteristics. These are major focuses of clinical and translational investigation. At the present time, until the results of the new USA Intergroup trial are available, surgery alone remains one standard of care. Chemoradiation therapy has been broadly accepted in the United States as being superior to radiation alone as a curative modality.

References

1. Blot WJ, Devesa SS, Kneller RW, Fraumeni JF (1991) Rising incidence of adenocarcinoma of the esophagus and gastric cardia. JAMA 265:1287–1289
2. Vokes EE (1993) Interactions of chemotherapy and radiation. Semin Oncol 20:70–79
3. Steel GG, Peckham MJ (1979) Exploitable mechanisms in combined radiotherapy-chemotherapy: the concept of additivity. Int J Radiat Onc Biol Phys 5:85–91
4. Lightdale C, Botet J, Brennan M et al (1989) Endoscopic ultrasonography compared to computerized tomography for preoperative staging of gastric cancer. Gastrointest Endosc 35:154 (abstract)
5. Tio TL, Coene PP, Luiken GJ, Tytgat GN (1990) Endosonography in the clinical staging of esophagogastric carcinoma. Gastrointest Endosc 36:s2–s10
6. Kelsen D, Ajani J, Ilson D, Daugherty K, Pazdur R (1994) A phase II trial of paclitaxel (Taxol) in advanced esophageal cancer: preliminary report. Semin Oncol 21:44–48
7. Roth JA, Pass HI, Flanagan MM, Graeber GM, Rosenberg JC, Steinberg S (1988) Randomized clinical trial of preoperative and postoperative adjuvant chemotherapy with cisplatin, vindesine, and bleomycin for carcinoma of the esophagus. J Thorac Cardiovasc Surg 96:242–248
8. Kelsen DP, Minsky B, Smith M et al (1990) Preoperative therapy for esophageal cancer: a randomized comparison of chemotherapy versus radiation therapy. J Clin Oncol 8:1352–1361
9. Nygaard K, Hagen S, Hansen HS et al (1992) Pre-operative radiotherapy prolongs survival in operable esophageal carcinoma: a randomized, multicenter study of pre-operative radiotherapy and chemotherapy. The second Scandinavian trial in esophageal cancer. World J Surg 16:1104–1110

Therapy of Cervical Esophageal Carcinoma

R. Roka, S. Kriwanek, S. Roka

First Surgical Department, Krankenanstalt Rudolfstiftung, Vienna, Austria

Abstract

Surgical treatment of cervical esophageal cancer is influenced by special problems arising from the anatomical characteristics of this organ. The cervical and thoracic extension of these tumors makes an extensive lymphadenectomy necessary, and radical resections often may only be achieved by laryngectomy. The extent of the resections performed determines the type of intestinal restoration by gastric or colonic interposition and small bowel transplantation. The patient's voice may be preserved by means of tracheopharyngeal shunts with intestinal interposition. The advances of radiation therapy and chemotherapy will enable less extended resections with greater rates of laryngeal preservation.

Introduction

Cancer of the cervical esophagus occurs rarely, but treatment remains a challenging surgical problem and demands special knowledge of abdominal, thoracic, and neck surgery. Unfortunately, the majority of these tumors are locally advanced. The main aim of treatment is therefore preservation or restoration of the voice rather than oncologically adequate resection.

Extent of Resection

The extent of the resection and the length of the tumor-free margins are issues of discussion mainly for thoracic cancer, but also for cervical cancer of the esophagus. Since the investigations carried out by Akiyama et al. [1] in the 1970s, intraepithelial, subepithelial, and intramural spread is a well-known fact. In general, a 5-cm tumor-free resection margin is required. More detailed recommendations have been made by Tsutsui et al. [11], who stated that a 3-cm margin is acceptable for T1 and T2 tumors, but that there is a 5% risk of accessory lesions remaining beyond the resection line. Conse-

Recent Results in Cancer Research, Vol. 155

quently, a segmental resection might be possible in selected patients depending on tumor stage and macroscopic appearance. In principle, according to a strict oncological concept, adequate resection includes cervical esophagolaryngo-pharyngectomy and transhiatal extraction of the thoracic esophagus as a routine procedure.

This correlates with our own experience. All six patients refusing laryngectomy developed local recurrences between 2 and 17 months (Table 1) after segmental resection of the cervical esophagus.

Three special techniques to lengthen the specimen proximal to the lesion have been published: temporary transection of the trachea facilitating tumor dissection [5], resection of the cricoid cartilage, and postcricoid mucosa dissection [10].

At present, there is an increasing tendency for more conservative surgery and larynx preservation based on improved preoperative treatment. This concept has to be investigated in further studies, and oncological rules have not yet been clearly defined.

Extent of Lymph Node Dissection

There is agreement about the high incidence of metastasis, but only a few investigations have been carried out, especially on thoracic involvement [6, 7, 12] (Table 2). Bilateral neck dissection plus the extirpation of the upper mediastinal nodes (group 100–106 according to the Japanese Cancer Society) seems to be an adequate compromise. More extensive lymph node surgery requires a three-field dissection. This would be associated with increased postoperative

Table 1. Tumor recurrence after segmental resections of the cervical esophagus

Tumor stage	Personal experiences (*n*)	Recurrence (months)
T2	2	11, 17
T3	4	2, 11, 13, 14

Table 2. Lymph node involvement

Tumor site	Involvement (%)	Reference
Paratracheal	32.0	[6]
Upper jugular	14.0	[6]
Middle jugular	18.0	[6]
Lower jugular	18.0	[6]
Posterior triangle	4.5	[6]
Paratracheal	71.4	[12]
Regional	50–70	
Mediastinal	32.0	[7]
Abdominal	0.0	[7]

morbidity and mortality rates. Furthermore, thoracic lymph node involvement originating from a cervical lesion may be sufficiently controlled by local treatment such as surgery only in a small number of patients.

The best approach for the cervicomediastinal part of the operation is a U-shaped cervical incision with a partial sternotomy and transverse lengthening in the third or fourth intercostal space.

Preservation of Parathyroid Function

Postoperative persistent hypocalcemia is an important factor impairing the patient's quality of life. In accordance with the authors' endocrine experience, one gland with a good blood supply is enough to guarantee sufficient parathyroid function. We therefore recommend leaving one upper gland together with a small rim of the thyroid bed and transplanting a second one.

Reconstruction

For reconstruction, interposition of the stomach with a pharyngogastric anastomosis is the operation performed most often. This procedure offers a number of advantages. It is a simple method, the stomach has a reliable blood supply, and only one anastomosis is necessary.

In contrast, the use of the colon has some disadvantages. It needs time-consuming preparation with three anastomoses and frequently a widening of the thoracic inlet by bone resection.

Furthermore, the colon is susceptible to complications. On the other hand, the advantages are the greater length of the organ and the possibility of voice restoration with a simple method to create a tracheopharyngeal shunt (Figs. 1, 2).

One of the advantages of a small bowel intestinal graft is the reliable peristalsis even after denervation [8]. This is an important benefit in patients in which there is preservation of the larynx, high anastomosis, and risk of aspiration. The jejunum is also suitable for small defects at distant sites where pedicled organs cannot be used, e.g., reoperations after complications or tumor recurrence [3].

We used a jejunal graft in situations with pharyngeal or esophageal defects or for voice restoration with a relatively low complication rate (Table 3).

Restoration of the Voice

Three methods for voice rehabilitation after pharyngolaryngo-esophagectomy exist: (1) artificial larynx, an external amplifier which most patients do not like to use; (2) a voice prosthesis, often complicated by chronic aspiration and poor functional results; and (3) a tracheopharyngeal shunt.

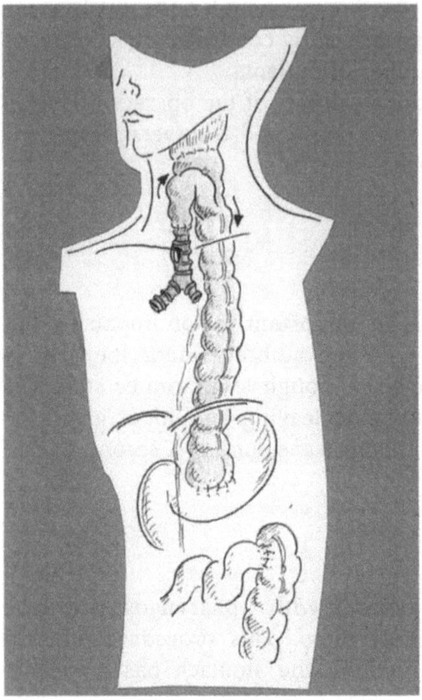

Fig. 1.

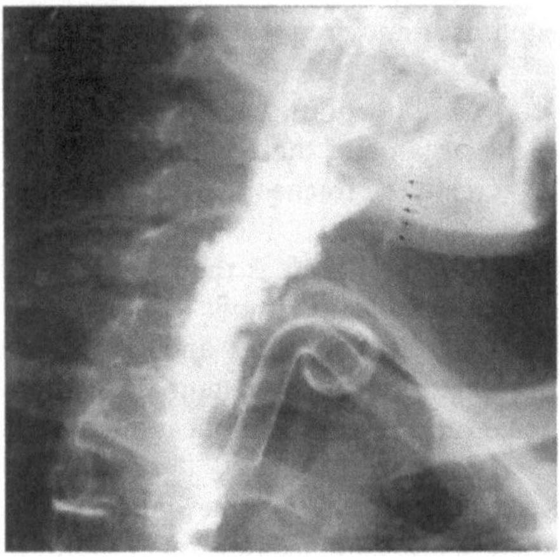

Fig. 2.

In the 1980s, we developed a tracheopharyngeal shunt with the interposition of a jejunal loop for patients who had undergone laryngectomy [9]. When the patient occludes the tracheostoma, the intestinal loop works like an air chamber and patients are able to speak with their own breath. Aspiration is prevented by the design and the peristalsis of the loop. The functional results are good. The maximal phonation time is 8.3 s; the voice is adequate for everyday purposes, and social verbal communication is possible.

Table 3. Reconstruction of cervical esophageal and pharyngeal defects in the transplanted small bowel. Jejunal graft, Vienna Study Group (1985–1996) (*n*, 93)

Jejunal graft	Patients (*n*)
Oropharynx	21
Hypopharynx	51
Cervical esophagus after laryngectomy	21
Patch	18
Tube	75
Necrosis	6 (6.4%)
Mortality	3 (3.2%)

This principle is also applicable after pharyngo-laryngo-esophagectomy by using the right colon for reconstruction. The colon is mobilized using several centimeters of the distal ileum. Care must be taken to preserve the arcade of the middle colic vessels. In the case of an early branching after their origin from the superior mesenteric vessels, we perform an auxiliary anastomosis between the ileocolic and cervical vessels. The cecum is anastomosed to the pharynx and the ileum to the tracheal stump (Fig. 1). Aspiration is prevented by the peristalsis of the ileum and the ileocecal valve, as shown by the postoperative X-ray examination (Fig. 2)

Tracheal Resection

In the literature, two authors have presented larger series of patients with resections of the trachea and mediastinal tracheostomy in tumors invading the trachea [2, 4]. This procedure cannot be recommended because of the high complication rate, short survival time, and poor quality of life. As recommended to reduce laryngectomy rates in general, these patients should be the focus of improved preoperative treatment.

References

1. Akiyama H, Ushiyama K, Kogure T (1971) Intraepithelial carcinoma associated with esophageal carcinoma. J Abd Surg 13(8):178–187
2. Burstein FD, Calcaterra TC (1987) Pectoralis flap – use in surgery of the lower neck and superior mediastinum. Arch Otolaryngol Head Neck Surg 113:73–77
3. Hermann M, Piza-Katzer H, Leitgeb A, Roka S, Roka R (1998) Palliation of anastomotic tumor recurrence after esophagectomy and gastric transposition: cervico-mediastinal resection and reconstruction by using a free jejunal transplant. Dis Esoph 11:1–3
4. Kato H, Tachimori Y, Watanabe H, Nakatsuka T, Mashima K, Ebihara S, Harii K (1994) Mediastinal tracheostomy during esophagectomy for cervicothoracic esophageal carcinoma invading the proximal trachea. J Surg Oncology 55:78–83
5. Kato H, Ebihara S (1992) Temporary transection of the trachea in cervical esophagectomy. Eur J Surg Oncol 18:335–339

6. Kelley DJ, Wolf R, Shaha AR, Spiro RH, Bains MS, Kraus DH, Shah JP (1995) Impact of clinicopathologic parameters on patient survival in carcinoma of the cervical esophagus. Am J Surg 170:427–431
7. Peracchia A, Bardini R, Ruol A, Segalin A, Castoro C, Asolati M, Tiso E (1990) Surgical management of carcinoma of the hypopharynx and cervical esophagus. Hepatogastroenterology 37:371–375
8. Roka R, Piza H (1982) Untersuchungen zur mechanischen Aktivität frei transplantierter Dünndarmabschnitte beim Hund. Acta Chir Austr 14:63–69
9. Roka R, Piza-Katzer H, Niederle B, Hausmaninger C, Grasl MCh (1990) Rekonstruktion von Defekten des Pharynx und des zervikalen Oesophagus. In: Langhans P, Schreiber HW, Häring R, Reding R, Siewert JR, Bünte H (Hrsg) Aktuelle Therapie des Oesophaguskarzinoms. Springer, Berlin Heidelberg New York, p 241–251
10. Stafford FW, Mathias DB (1986) Pharyngectomy for post-cricoid carcinoma with preservation of the larynx. J Laryngol Otol 100:1385–1398
11. Tsutsui S, Kuwano H, Watanabe M, Kitamura M, Sugimachi K (1995) Resection margin for squamous cell carcinoma of the esophagus. Ann Surg 222(2):193–202
12. Weber RS, Marvel J, Smith P, Hankins P, Wolf P, Goepfert H (1993) Paratracheal lymph node dissection for carcinoma of the larynx, hypopharynx and cervical esophagus. Otolaryngol Head Neck Surg 108(1):11–17

Esophageal Cancer: A European Perspective

A. Peracchia [1], L. Bonavina [1], A. Ruol [2], H. Stein [3]

[1] Istituto di Chirurgia Generale e Oncologia Chirurgica, University of Milan, Ospedale Maggiore, I.R.C.C.S., Via F. Sforza 35, I-20122 Milano, Italy
[2] Istituto di Chirurgia Generale, University of Padova, Italy
[3] Chirurgische Klinik und Poliklinik, Klinikum rechts der Isar der TU München, Ismaningerstr. 22, D-81675 Munich, Germany

Abstract

A survey was conducted among a group of European surgeons in order to investigate current attitudes and strategies in the management of squamous cell carcinoma of the esophagus. The survey consisted of a questionnaire mailed to surgeons in eight different countries with extensive clinical experience and scientific interest in the field. Eight questionnaires including the data of 6146 operated patients were available for analysis. A consensus emerged among the panelists that protocols of induction therapy should be routinely used in patients with locally advanced disease, especially in supracarinal tumors. Four of the surgeons advocated bilateral neck dissection in these patients. A progressive improvement in survival over the past three decades was noted. After 1990, the postoperative mortality rate was 6.2% after surgery alone and 9.7% after chemoradiation therapy followed by surgery. The 5-year survival rate after a complete resection was 38.5%. In the opinion of the panelists, esophagectomy remains the "gold standard" of therapy and should be regarded as an integral component of the treatment plan for patients with squamous cell carcinoma.

Introduction

Esophageal cancer remains one of the most difficult malignancies to treat, since in the Western world patients usually present with advanced disease and cure is not a realistic goal in this situation [1]. Although generally considered to be a relatively uncommon disease, esophageal cancer is the ninth most frequent cancer and the sixth most frequent cause of death from cancer worldwide. The burden of esophageal cancer in terms of morbidity and mortality varies greatly according to the geographic area. In Europe, highest incidence rates are found in France for males and in Scotland for females. Over the last decade, the incidence of esophageal cancer has sharply increased in Hungary in both men and women [2, 3]. Besides these geographical changes, a major shift in histological type has been reported in the United Kingdom and Denmark, resulting in a sharp increase in adenocarcinoma [4].

A major literature review by Earlam and Cunha-Melo [5] revealed a 29% mortality rate and a mean 5-year survival of 4% after surgical therapy for esophageal cancer. Based on these data, the authors concluded that esophagectomy had the "highest operative mortality of any routinely performed surgical procedure today." This article had a profound impact on the approach to the disease until another major literature review by Muller et al. [6] reversed the predominant pessimistic attitude toward esophageal carcinoma and esophageal surgery.

The aim of the present study was to assess and compare the current strategies in the treatment of squamous cell carcinoma of the esophagus adopted in some referral centers for this disease in Western Europe.

Methods

In October 1997, a questionnaire was devised by the first author and mailed to seven European surgeons with proven clinical experience and scientific interest in the field. There were 19 questions dealing with the following issues: the role of preoperative chemoradiation therapy in relation to the stage and anatomical site of the tumor; the optimal surgical strategy for supra- and infracarinal tumors; the use of minimally invasive procedures; the extension of lymphadenectomy; and the use of adjuvant therapy after curative or palliative resection. In addition, the panel was asked about the immediate and long-term results of treatment during three different periods of time: before 1980, between 1984 and 1989, and since 1990.

Results

Eight questionnaires (including the one compiled in the first author's own institution) were examined. The data of 6146 surgically treated patients were analyzed.

There was a consensus among the panelists about the need for neoadjuvant chemoradiation in patients with locally advanced tumors (T3–T4). Half of the surgeons believed that the same treatment should be applied to tumors less advanced but located above the carina. One of the surgeons believed that this kind of preoperative treatment should be reserved only for patients included in randomized studies, regardless of stage and location. According to three of the surgeons, the presence of metastatic nodes represents an indication for preoperative therapy independent of the T parameter.

The majority of the panelists believed that the ideal surgical approach for supracarinal tumors is a right thoracotomy followed by laparotomy and cervicotomy. As far as infracarinal tumors are concerned, the approach preferred by half of the surgeons consists of a laparotomy followed by right thoracotomy. Esophagectomy without thoracotomy is reserved for selected patients. There was a consensus among panelists that esophageal dissection through thoracoscopy does not have any role in the surgical therapy; however, three surgeons believed that it may be reasonable to mobilize the stomach through laparoscopy.

The majority of the surgeons believed that lymphadenectomy should also include the upper mediastinal nodes in supracarinal tumors; however, only four of the panelists advocated bilateral neck dissection in these patients. Five surgeons believed that adjuvant therapy is indicated after R0 resection when more than 20% of the nodes are involved.

Analysis of data provided by the panelists showed a decrease in hospital mortality rates from 14.1% (range, 12%–15%) before 1980 to 5.7% (range, 1.4%–10%) between 1984 and 1989; the mortality rate since 1990 is 6.2% (range, 1.5%–11%). The mean postoperative mortality rate was 9.7% (range, 3.5%–16%) in patients treated with neoadjuvant chemoradiation therapy. The mean overall 5-year survival rate after R0 resection was 17.5%, 31.5%, and 38.5%, respectively, during the three periods under review.

Comment

This survey was conducted to assess the current status of treatment of squamous cell esophageal cancer in leading European surgical institutions. The aim was not to have a literature review, but updated comments from opinion leaders in the field using data from patients treated in their own centers.

The first important message emerging from this study is that most centers are now using protocols of induction therapy for treating squamous cell esophageal carcinoma. Based on clinical T staging, most centers favor induction therapy for T3–T4 tumors and use these regimens on a routine basis, especially in supracarinal tumors. The opinions of the panelists confirm the conclusions of the 1995 ISDE Consensus Conference, which suggested first-line chemoradiotherapy in patients with a locally advanced, non-metastatic squamous cell carcinoma of the esophagus [7].

Another major finding of this study was that, in dedicated centers, the mortality rate after esophagectomy is now about 5%. After a complete (R0) resection, a 5-year survival rate of more than 35% is to be expected. Routine mediastinal lymphadenectomy extended to the apex of the chest was considered beneficial by the majority of the surgeons participating in this survey. The value of cervical lymphadenectomy remains investigational; however, half of the panelists advocated bilateral neck dissection for patients with supracarinal tumors.

Conclusions

Complete surgical resection remains the mainstay of treatment in squamous cell esophageal carcinoma. During the 1990s, surgical mortality in esophageal cancer patients has considerably declined and the 5-year survival rate has improved. Today, the multimodal approach is becoming increasingly accepted. In the future, it may become the therapeutic strategy of choice even in patients with potentially resectable infracarinal tumors. It is likely that current prospective studies involving neoadjuvant regimens will offer the best hope of improving survival rates. International registries are urgently needed to coordinate efforts to further improve results.

Acknowledgements. This study was made possible by the participation of J.M. Collard (Brussels), F. Fékété (Paris), B. Launois (Rennes), T. Lerut (Leuven), J. Mendes de Almeida (Lisbon), R. Siewert (Munich), and A. Watson (London).

Supported by F.I.R.C./Fondazione Italiana per la Ricerca sul Cancro.

References

1. Bonavina L (1995) Early oesophageal cancer. Results of a European multicenter survey. Br J Surg 82:98–101
2. Munoz N, Castellsagué X (1994) Epidemiology of oesophageal cancer. Eur J Gastroenterol Hepatol 6:649–655
3. Murray C, Lopez A (1997) Mortality by cause for eight regions of the world: global burden of disease study. Lancet 349:1269–1276
4. Macfarlane G, Boyle P (1994) The epidemiology of oesophageal cancer in the UK and other European countries. J R Soc Med 87:334–337
5. Earlam R, Cunha-Melo J (1980) Oesophageal squamous-cell carcinoma. A critical review of surgery. Br J Surg 67:381–390
6. Muller J, Erasmi H, Stelzner M, Zieren U, Pichlmaier H (1990) Surgical therapy of oesophageal carcinoma. Br J Surg 77:845–857
7. Ruol A, panel of experts (1996) Multimodality treatment for non-metastatic cancer of the thoracic esophagus. Dis Esoph 9 [Suppl 1]:39–54

Significance of Extended Systemic Lymph Node Dissection for Thoracic Esophageal Carcinoma in Japan

H. Watanabe, H. Kato, Y. Tachimori

Department of Surgery, National Cancer Center Hospital, 1-1, Tsukiji 5-Chome, Chuo-ku, Tokyo, 104-0045 Japan

Abstract

In 1986, several institutions in Japan began to employ extensive lymphadenectomy for thoracic esophageal cancer. The aim of this article is to point out several confusing factors concerning the use of the terms "tow-field" and "three-field" lymph node dissection for thoracic esophageal cancer. In two-field nodal dissection, two components are included with (modern two-field) or without (traditional two-field) nodal dissection around both recurrent laryngeal nerve chains in the upper mediastinum. We studied a series of 353 patients resected for thoracic esophageal cancer in our institution. The patients were divided into three groups. Group A was the traditional two-field group of patients who underwent thoracoabdominal lymphadenectomy without upper mediastinal lymph node dissection after preoperative irradiation; group B was the modern two-field group, with additional upper mediastinal lymph node dissection; and group C was the three-field group with additional neck lymph node dissection. Groups B and C were operated on during the same period and did not received preoperative irradiation. The 5-year survival rate in group B was 54.9%, which was better than the 47.6% rate after three-field dissection (group C). The key to extensive lymphadenectomy for thoracic esophageal cancer does not lie in "cervical dissection" but in the meticulous dissection of the lymph nodes around the right and left recurrent laryngeal nerves.

Introduction

Many Japanese surgeons perform wide lymphadenectomy as a curative operation for thoracic esophageal cancer. From 1962 to 1984, we routinely dissected middle and lower mediastinal and abdominal lymph nodes in our radical operation after preoperative irradiation. However, the 5-year survival rate of these patients remained at around 20–25% [1]. Based on the first clinical description of cervical lymph node metastasis of thoracic esophageal

Recent Results in Cancer Research, Vol. 155

cancer by Sannohe and coworkers in 1980 [2], many Japanese surgeons performed a trial of neck lymph node dissection with total mediastinal and abdominal dissection. As reported in the literature [3–5], there have been various trials concerning the effect of cervical lymph adenectomy, although they do not include any strictly randomized trials. From detecting metastatic lymph nodes in the neck during nodal neck dissection and on the basis of historical studies, most Japanese surgeons assumed that lymph node dissection in the neck would improve the prognosis of thoracic esophageal cancer. Nevertheless, the prerequisites for comparative studies after different modes of lymph node dissection had not been clarified. We compited a list of prerequisites; our thoracic surgeons were then divided into two groups, and we started comparative studies concerning the different types of lymph node dissection to clarify the essential factors in effective extensive lymphadenectomy.

Material and Methods

A total of 353 patients with thoracic esophageal carcinoma underwent esophagectomy and lymphadenectomy during two different periods (Fig. 1). From February 1982 to December 1985, 114 patients received incomplete nodal dissection in the upper mediastinum combinded with preoperative irradiation (traditional two-field). The second and third groups consisted of 239 patients who received extended lymph node dissection around both recurrent laryngeal nerves without preoperative irradiation from January 1988 to December 1994. The patients undergoing operations from January 1986 to December 1988 were excluded from this study, because the operative technique of nodal dissection was not standardized. In the second group, modern

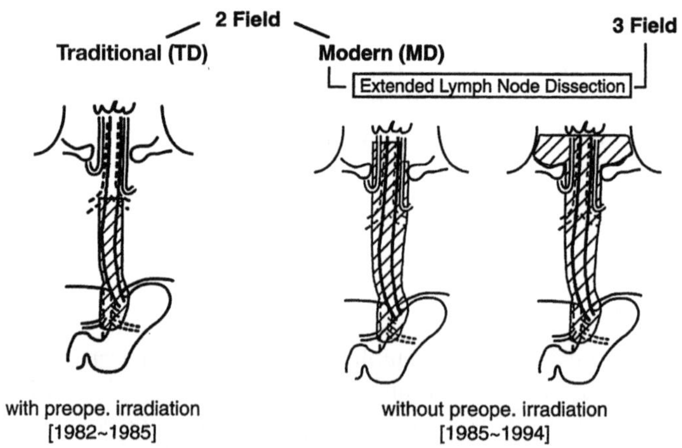

Fig. 1 a–c. Different types of lymph node dissection for thoracic esophageal cancer in Japan. **a** Traditional two-field with preoperative irradiation (1982–1985). **b** Modern two-field and **c** three-field extended lymph node dissection without preoperative irradiation (1985–1994)

Table 1. Type of nodal dissection procedure

Procedure	Patients (*n*)	Time period
Traditional two-field	114	1982–1985
Modern two-field[a]	98	1988–1994
Three-field[a]	141	

[a] Extended lymph node dissection; upper thoracic esophageal carcinoma was excluded.

two-field dissection, the mediastinal approach alone without neck dissection, was performed ($n=98$). In the third group (three-field dissection), the cervical lymph nodes, including the subclavicular lymph node, were removed by the cervical approach (Table 1). These patients were assigned to thoracic surgeons randomly. One surgeon performed the modern two-field operation, and two other surgeons performed three-field operations. We analyzed the survival rates according to the different types of nodal dissection. Table 1 shows the procedures used in the two different periods. The survival rates were computed according to the life-table method of Culter and Ederar. Patients who died of operative complications were excluded. The differences between survival curves were analyzed by the generalized Wilcoxon method and long-rank test.

Results

Before analyzing survival data, we clarified the prerequisites for comparative studies after lymph node dissection as follows:

1. Upper thoracic esophageal cancer should be excluded. Because of the upward flow in the upper esophagus, cervical lymphadenectomy is obligatory for these lesions.
2. In different precedures, the grade of lymph node dissection in the upper mediastinum (especially around both recurrent laryngeal nerves) must be similar.
3. The surgical technique in both procedures must be consistent.

Variation in Frequency of Lymph Node Metastasis According to the Area Dissected

Up to 1982, we did not dissect the lymph nodes around the recurrent laryngeal nerve chain in the upper mediastinum, instead performing preoperative irradiation. Beginning in 1986, we started dissecting lymph nodes in this field on a regular basis. The change in lymph node dissection increased the recognition of the frequency of upper mediastinal lymph node metastasis from 40.9% to 66.7%, as shown in Table 2. Before 1986, we only removed the

Table 2. Frequency of lymph node metastasis according to different type of nodal dissection

Lymph node groups	Positive rate of metastasis (%)	
	Traditional two-field	Modern two- and three-field
Upper mediastinum	40.9	66.7
Middle and lower mediastinum	51.4	56.3
Paracardia	57.1	54.9
Agastric sinistra and celiac trunk	33.3	38.0

lymph nodes in the upper mediastinum without paying much attention to lymph nodes around the recurrent laryngeal nerve (traditional two-field group). However, the grade of lymph node dissection in other regions except for the upper mediastinum is similar to that of modern two-field groups.

Target and Approach of Lymph Node Dissection

At present, cervicothoracic and upper mediastinal dissection is carried out via thoracotomy from the right fourth or fifth intercostal space with the patient in the left lateral position. The most important procedure is lymph node dissection around the right and left recurrent laryngeal nerve. There is no borderline between the neck and upper mediastinum, as shown in Fig. 2.

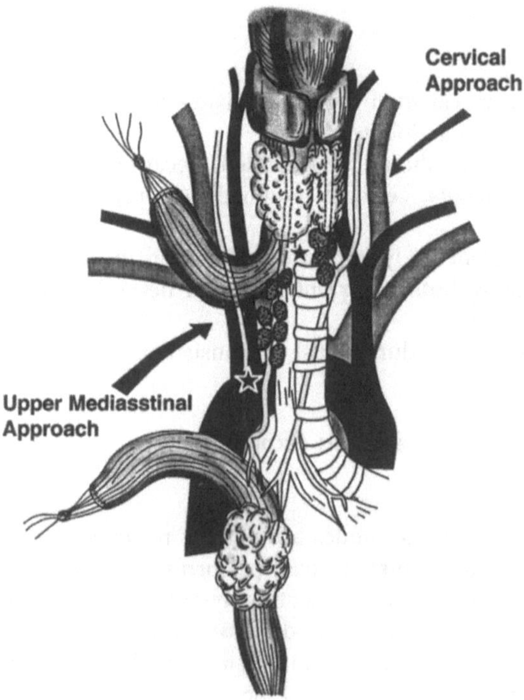

Fig. 2. Target and approach of lymph node dissection for thoracic esophageal cancer: lymph node around the right and left recurrent laryngeal nerve

There are two approaches to lymph node dissection around recurrent laryngeal nerve, one from the upper mediastinal and the other from the upper mediastinum and neck. The lymph nodes around recurrent laryngeal nerve chains of the upper mediastinal and of the neck should be considered as one entity. In the procedure from the upper mediastinum and neck, additional dissection of bilateral subclavicular nodes, deep cervical nodes, and internal juglar nodes is performed.

Long-Term Results According to the Different Series and Procedures of Lymph Nodes Dissection

The overall survival curve was better in the modern two-field and three-field groups. The 5-year survival rate in patients undergoing modern two-field lymph node dissection was 54.9% (1990–94), 47.6% (1985–89), and which was significantly better ($p<0.001$) than the 22.8% achieved using the traditional two-field approach, as shown in Fig. 3.

A comparison of survical rates between patients in whom the primary lesion was located in the middle thoracic esophaus who underwent two- or three-field dissection is shown in Fig. 4. A tendency for better survival was noted with the modern two-field dissection, but this was not significant. As shown in Fig. 5, a comparison of the survival curves in the modern two-field and three-field lymph node dissection groups for lower thoracic and abdominal esophageal cancer also showed essentially no difference between the two groups.

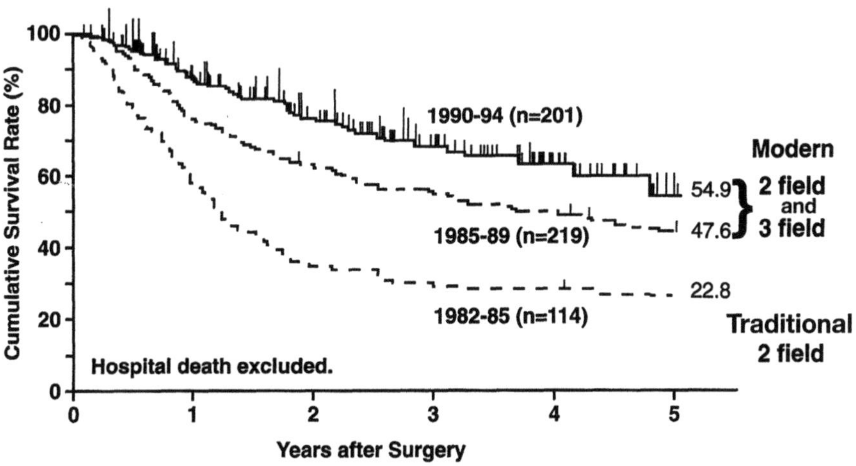

Fig. 3. Comparison of survival curves in the different series and different procedures of lymph node dissection. *Top curve*, modern two-field and three-field approach, 1990–1994 ($n=201$). *Middle curve*, modern two-field and three-field approach, 1985–1989 ($n=219$). *Botton curve*, traditional two-field approach, 1982–1985 ($n=114$). Hospital deaths excluded

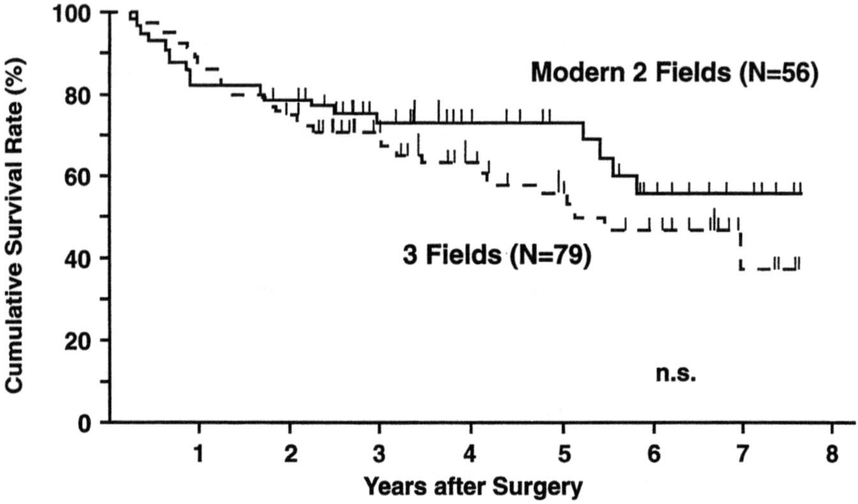

Fig. 4. Comparison of survival curves for modern two-field (*solid-line*, *n*=56) and three-field lymph node dissection (*dashed line*, *n*=79) for midthoracic esophageal cancer. The difference was not significant

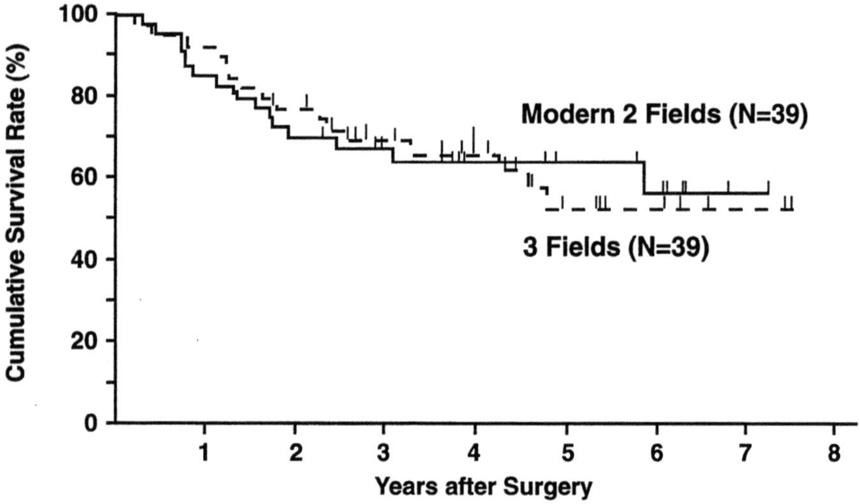

Fig. 5. Comparison of survival curves for modern two-field (*solid-line*, n=39) and three-field lymph node dissection (*dashed line*, *n*=39) for lower thoracic and abdominal esophageal cancer

Key Factor in Extended Lymphadenectomy

From the analysis performed by comparing the survival rates achieved using modern two-field and three-field lymph node dissection it can be seen that essential factor in extended lymphadenectomy does not lie in cervical dissec-

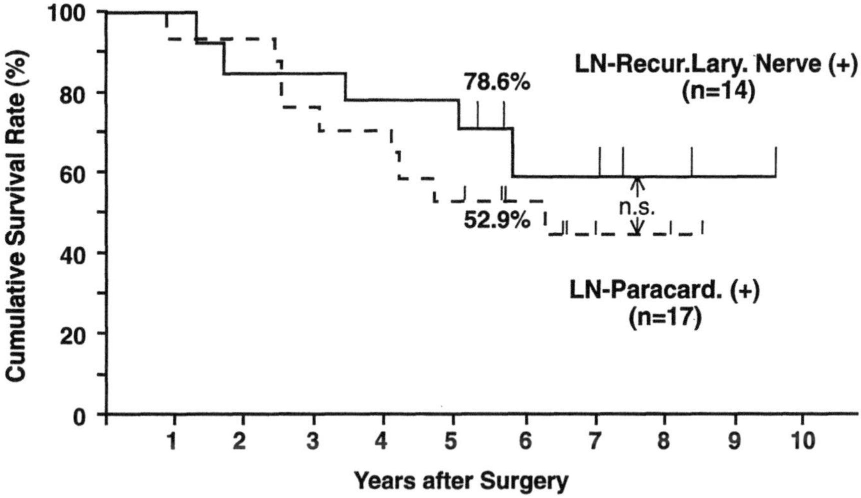

Fig. 6. Comparison of survical curves in patients with single metastasis to the lymph node around recurrent laryngeal nerve (*solid line*, $n = 14$) and paracadia (*dashed line*, $n = 17$)

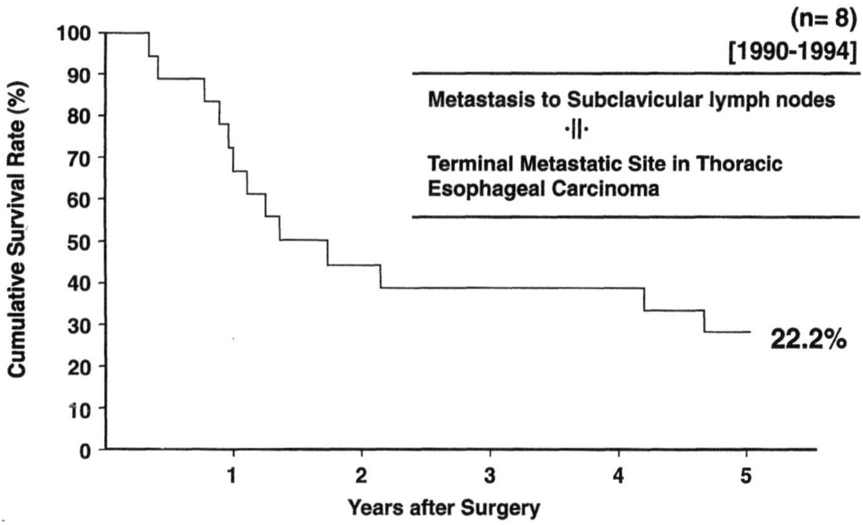

Fig. 7. Survical curve in patients with metastases to the subclavicular lymph nodes removed by three-field nodal dissection from 1990 to 1994 ($n = 8$)

tion. The question therefore arises as to the importance of the lymph nodes around the right and left recurrent laryngel nerves. As shown in Fig. 6, the 5-year survival rate in patients with single lymph node metastasis around the right or left recurrent laryngeal nerves was 78.6%, and this long-term result was similar to that of patients with single metastasis of paracardiac lymph nodes. The good prognosis in patients with metastasic nodes around the recurrent laryngeal nerve suggests that this node may be the first site in the process of nodal metastasis for thoracic esophageal cancers. On the other hand, the 5-year survival rate in patients with single metastasis to subclavicular lymph nodes removed by three-field lymph node dissection was 22.2% (Fig. 7). The key to extended (modern two-field or three-field) lymphadenectomy does not lie in total cervical dissection (neck dissection), but in the dissection of lymph nodes around the recurrent laryngeal nerves (upper mediastinum).

Presence of Micrometastasis in Fibrofatty Tissue According to the Site of the Lymph Node

As an additional fact or suggesting the superiority of extended lymphadenectomy in the upper mediastinum, there may be extranodal lymphatic vessel infiltration, i.e., micrometastasis, in fibrofatty tissue around lymph nodes (Table 3). As shown in Table 4, the frequency of micrometastasis was high (27.3% in the tissue around the upper mediastinal lymph nodes). In contrast, the frequency at the neck is very low (only 3.0%). These findings emphasize the value of extended lymphadenectomy in the upper mediastinum for potentially curable esophageal cancers [6].

Differences in Mode of Postoperative Recurrence Between Modern Two-Field and Three-Field Dissection

In terms of the frequency of lymph node recurrence, the patients who underwent three-field dissection showed higher recurrent rates than patients who underwent modern two-field dissection (Table 4). This difference was statistically significant. The difference between the two groups in the rate of organ recurrence was not significant.

Table 3. Rate of micrometastasis (extranodal lymphatic vessel permeation) and node metastasis according to site of lymph node in 77 patients

Site of lymph node	Rate of micrometastasis (%)	Rate of node metastasis (%)
Neck	3.0	18.0
Upper mediastinum	27.3	38.9
Middle mediastinum	18.1	36.4
Lower mediastinum	12.1	28.5
Paracardia	21.2	62.3

Table 4. Postoperative mode of recurrence after lymph node dissection (1986–1989)

Dissection procedure	Lymph node positive		Lymph node negative		Organ positive		Organ negative	
	(*n*)	(%)	(*n*)	(%)	(*n*)	(%)	(*n*)	(%)
Modern two-field (*n*=23)	7	30.4	16	69.6*	17	73.9	6	26.1**
Three-field (*n*=32)	20	62.5	12	37.5*	16	50.0	16	50.0**

* $p < 0.05$; ** not significant.

Discussion

Thoracic esophageal cancer metastasizes in a stepwise fashion. More lymphatic vessels run longitudinally than horizontally in the esophageal submucosal layer, and distant nodal metastasis therefore appears relatively early in patients with esophageal cancer. Because of this, extensive and systemic lymph node dissection is needed to improve the prognosis after surgical treatment. Based on the first clinical description of cervical lymph node metastasis of thoracic esophageal cancer by Sannohe in 1980 [2], many Japanese surgeons perform cervicothoracic, abdominal (three-field) lymphadenectomy as a curative operation. As reported in the literature [3–5], there have been various trials concerning the effect of cervical lymphadenectomy in thoracic esophageal cancer, although they have not included any strictly randomized trials. There are many problems with nonrandomized studied, including the following:

1. Most trials are retrospective and uncontrolled historical studies.
2. In the so-called two-field group, some authors reported the traditional two-field group (only pick-up dissection of the lymph nodes in upper mediastinum) and the modern two-field group (extended lymphadenectomy in the upper mediastinum) together. The frequency of upper mediastinal lymph node metastasis therefore increases from 40.9% to 66.7%, as shown in Table 2.
3. The extent of nodal dissection in the upper mediastinum is different between the two-field and three-field lymphadenectomy group in almost all reports in the literature in Japan.
4. Most trials do not exclude upper esophageal cancer. In ordinary lymphadenectomy for upper esophageal cancer, it is only reasonable to dissect the cervical lymph nodes.
5. The survival curves in most reports are cumulative, not actuarial, and are difficult to compare.

The terms "two-field" and "three-field" can cause confusion because the former includes both the traditional two-field and the modern two-field approach. We have been resecting middle or lower mediastinal and abdominal lymph nodes (traditional two-field) since 1982. After the introduction of this operation, recurrenct disease most often oncurred in the upper mediastinal and the neck lymph nodes. We tried the extended lymphadenectomy around the area of the recurrent laryngeal nerve from a mediastinal or cervical approach to evaluate the safety of the procedure. In January 1986, we began the present trial to evaluate the effectiveness of extended lymphadenectomy either from the mediastinal or the cervical approach. From January 1986 to December 1989, our extended lymphadenectomy technique in 219 patients was not standardized, but from January 1990 to December 1994, a standard technique was employed. Beginning in 1986, we compared the two methods of extended lymphadenectomy. The overall operative 5-year survival rate of 54.9% in the latest series (1990–1994) seems satisfactory compared with that of current reports [5, 7]. Our latest overall 5-year survival rate of 54.9% is as high as that reported by Akiyama and colleagues [5]. The operation time is approximately 120 min longer in the three-field group than in the modern two-field group.

Neither the average operative blood loss nor the rate of postoperative pneumonia or anastomotic leakage differed significantly between the two groups. However, the main complication after three-field operations was bleeding from a large vessel of the neck combined with wound infection at the neck, and disseminated recurrent cancer appeared early in the neck. Although our two groups of patients were operated on by two different groups of surgeons, the surgeons had been working together in the same institution and performed the procedure with comparable skill. One surgeon performing modern two-field lymphadenectomy had 30 years of experience, and the other two surgeons performing three-field lymphadenectomy had 15 and 20 years of experience respectively. Our controlled comparison of survival between the modern two-field procedure and the three-field procedure did not show any superiority for the three-field group. In both arms, the grade of dissection in the upper mediastinum was similar. The key to extended lymphadenectomy for thoracic esphageal cancer does not lie in wide cervical dissection, but in the dissection of the nodes around the right and left recurrent laryngeal nerve. Even if the subclavicular lymph nodes are metastatic in patients with middle- and lower thoracic esophageal cancer, the removal of these lymph nodes does not seem to extend the long-term survival.

References

1. Akakura I, Nakamura Y, Kakegawa T et al (1970) Surgery of carcinoma of the esophagus with preoperative radiation. Chest 57 (1):47–57
2. Sannohe Y, Hirazuka R, Doki K (1980) Behavior and treatment of cervical lymph node metastasis for thoracic esophageal cancer (in Japanese). J Jpn Assoc Thorac Surg 28:241–247
3. Isono K, Sato H, Nakayama K (1991) Results of a nationwide study on the three-field lymph node dissection of esophageal cancer. Oncology 48:411–420

4. Kato H, Watanabe H, Tachimori R (1991) Evaluation of neck lymph node dissection for esophageal cancer. Oncology 48:411–420
5. Akiyama H, Tsurumaru H, Udagawa H et al (1994) Systemic lymph node dissection for esophageal cancer-effective or not? Dis Esophagus 7 (1):2–13
6. Watanabe H (1997) New targets of treatment for esophageal carcinoma: micrometastasis in the operative field. Ann Thorac Cardiovasc Surg 3(2):84–85
7. Sasaki K, Muto T, Tanaka O et al (1988) The significance of systemic lymphadenectomy for thoracic esophageal carcinoma. In: Siewert JR, Holsher AH (eds) Disease of the esophagus. Springer, Berlin Heidelberg New York, pp 687–690

Gastric Conditioning

J.D. Urschel

Department of Thoracic Surgery, Roswell Park Cancer Institute, Buffalo, New York, USA

Abstract

The etiology of esophagogastric anastomotic leaks is often multifactorial. However, occult ischemia of the gastric fundus is an important cause. In gastric conditioning, preliminary partial gastric devascularization is carried out 2–3 weeks before construction of the esophagogastric anastomoses. Gastric vascularity improves over this time. In animal studies, gastric conditioning has reduced the incidence of anastomotic leaks. Clinically, the concept of gastric conditioning can be used in several ways. Esophagectomy can be done at one stage, then a cervical esophagogastric anastomosis can be completed as a second-stage procedure. Pre-esophagectomy angiographic gastric artery embolization is another method of gastric conditioning. Finally, laparoscopic partial gastric devascularization can be done at the time of laparoscopic cancer staging. For gastric conditioning to be clinically useful, the benefit from reduction in leaks must be greater than the costs and morbidity of the conditioning procedure itself.

Introduction

Despite advances in operative technique and post-operative care, esophagectomy for esophageal cancer continues to be a relatively morbid surgical procedure. Esophagectomy for esophageal cancer has an operative mortality of approximately 10% [1]. Esophageal reconstruction is usually achieved by gastric transposition and esophagogastric anastomosis. Anastomotic leakage complicates 5%–20% of procedures [1–3]. Although pulmonary complications have surpassed anastomotic leaks as the leading cause of operative mortality in many modern esophagectomy series [4, 5], anastomotic leaks are still responsible for approximately one-third of operative deaths [6]. Elimination of anastomotic leaks would greatly reduce the morbidity and mortality of esophagectomy.

The etiology of esophagogastric anastomotic leaks is often multifactorial, but errors in surgical technique and occult ischemia of the gastric tube are

Recent Results in Cancer Research, Vol. 155

the two most important causes [2, 7, 8]. Good results have been reported for many different anastomotic techniques. Stapled anastomoses were once thought to be safer than hand-sewn anastomoses, but randomized trials have refuted this notion [6, 9, 10]. Surgical experience is a more critical determinant of success than the specific anastomotic technique used [7, 10, 11].

Gastric-Tube Ischemia

Mobilization of the stomach for gastric transposition requires division of the left gastric, left gastroepiploic, and short gastric arteries. Because the gastroepiploic arcade is infrequently complete [12], blood supply to the mobilized proximal stomach is largely derived from a rich submucosal plexus of vessels [13–15]. Although frank gangrene is rare if the stomach is properly mobilized [16], occult ischemia of the gastric fundus (tip of gastric tube) is often present [15]. This is a major factor in the genesis of esophagogastric anastomotic leaks [2, 7, 8, 15].

The importance of gastric-tube ischemia has been stressed by many investigators. Ischemia has been quantified by measuring gastric oxygenation (Clark electrode or oximetry), perfusion (laser-doppler flowmetry), blood flow (hydrogen clearance method), and tonometry. Miyoshi measured gastric-tube oxygenation in dogs and humans using a Clark electrode [17]. A PtO_2 of less than 30 mmHg was associated with a high incidence of anastomotic leaks. Jacobi measured gastric submucosal oxygenation with a Clark electrode in 20 patients undergoing esophagectomy [18]. Baseline PtO_2 was 55 mmHg. After stomach mobilization and creation of the gastric tube, PtO_2 fell to 26 mmHg. Two patients developed anastomotic leaks, but development of leak did not correlate with measured PtO_2. Abo reported gastric-tube PtO_2 values that were approximately 50% of baseline gastric values [19]. The occurrence of anastomotic leaks correlated with lower gastric-tube PtO_2 in this study. Cooper also studied changes in gastric-tissue oxygenation in patients undergoing esophagectomy [20]. With gastric mobilization, PtO_2 fell from a mean baseline value of 77 mmHg to a mean of 36 mmHg. Salo assessed gastric-tube oxygenation using a pulse oximeter and only constructed the anastomosis if oxygen saturation was over 84% [21]. If the saturation was lower, additional stomach was resected and oximetry was repeated. Using this approach, there were no anastomotic leaks in 16 patients.

Schilling measured gastric-tube perfusion in 11 patients using a laser-Doppler flowmeter [22]. Baseline gastric fundal tissue perfusion was 323 PU (perfusion units). It fell to 69 PU after creation of the gastric tube. Since no leaks occurred in these 11 patients, it was not possible to correlate anastomotic leaks with tissue perfusion. In a subsequent animal experiment, the same authors showed a trend toward a higher incidence of anastomotic leaks with poorer gastric-tube perfusion, but the correlation did not reach statistical significance [23]. Pierie used laser-Doppler flowmetry to measure gastric-tube perfusion in 30 patients undergoing esophagectomy [24]. Perfusion at the tip of the gastric tube dropped to 52% of baseline values. Three leaks occurred. Although perfusion values in these three patients were low, no perfusion value could be identified that significantly predicted the occurrence of leaks. However, perfusion measurements were useful in predicting occurrence of anastomotic strictures. Abo also measured gastric-tube perfusion with laser-Doppler flowmetry [19]. Patients with anastomotic leaks had significantly lower gastric-tube perfusion than those without leaks.

Sugimachi assessed various types of gastric tubes in dogs using hydrogen clearance calculation of blood flow [25]. Creating an excessively narrow (1.5 cm) gastric tube interrupted the submucosal vascular network and resulted in poor blood flow at the gastroplasty tip. Machens measured intramucosal pH (pHi) with a gastric tonometer in 12 esophagectomy patients [26]. The median pHi in patients with anastomotic leaks was lower than the pHi of patients without leaks.

Gastric-tube ischemia can result from systemic hypotension. Several investigators have emphasized the importance of maintaining adequate overall tissue perfusion after esophagectomy. In an animal experiment, intraoperative blood loss and hypotension were shown to be detrimental to esophagogastric anastomotic healing [27]. In a clinical study, oxygen delivery 6 h after esophagectomy was significantly higher in 86 patients without anastomotic leak than in 29 who had an anastomotic leak [28]. Retrospective clinical studies have identified excessive intra-operative blood loss, and resulting hypotension, as predisposing factors for esophagogastric anastomotic leakage [29, 30].

Gastric Conditioning: Physiology

In some respects, mobilization of the stomach for esophageal replacement is analogous to skin-flap transposition for cutaneous reconstruction [31]. In the past, when random arterial pattern skin flaps were mainstays of reconstructive surgery, flap necrosis was an all too common problem. To reduce the likelihood of skin-flap failure, reconstructive surgeons mobilized and partially devascularized flaps, then replaced them in their original position. The distal end of the flap often became ischemic, but its viability gradually improved as long as the additional stress of flap transposition and oxygen demands of wound healing were postponed. After a delay of approximately 2–3 weeks, the skin flap was transposed to its recipient bed. By delaying transposition, collateral vessels developed and flap vascularity improved. Flap necrosis and wound dehiscence were thereby reduced. In modern reconstructive surgery, the delay phenomenon has been the subject of renewed interest. The concept is now applied to muscle flaps [32].

Although the beneficial effects of delay phenomenon on flap vascularity and survival are widely appreciated by plastic surgeons [32–34], the physiological mechanisms of flap delay phenomenon are not completely understood [35]. Conditioning to ischemia is one possible mechanism to explain the delay phenomenon. "Conditioning" is a process of neovascularization, which occurs in response to ongoing ischemia within a tissue flap. Experimental studies support its importance in the delay process; the most ischemic parts of flaps show the greatest increase in vascularity over the delay period [36]. Another possible explanation for the beneficial effect of the delay phenomenon is altered microcirculatory flow from denervation [37, 38]. Finally, tissue wounding in of itself has an effect on tissue vascularity that is not specifically related to flap ischemia [39, 40].

Gastric Conditioning: Laboratory Studies

Gastric conditioning and its effect on anastomotic healing have been studied in the rat. Since the stomach, as opposed to the esophagus, is the potential ischemic element in esophagogastrostomy anastomoses [41, 42], a model was initially developed to study the effect of ischemia and gastric conditioning on gastric anastomotic healing [43]. The degree of ischemia created in this rat model simulated that seen with gastric mobilization for esophageal replacement in humans [17, 18, 22, 24]. Partial gastric devascularization impaired gastric anastomotic wound healing [44]. The detrimental effect of devascularization on gastric tissue perfusion was partly ameliorated by a 2-week period of gastric conditioning [43]. Gastric conditioning reduced the incidence of gastric anastomotic leaks [45, 46] and increased anastomotic wound-breaking strength [45].

Gastric conditioning has been shown to improve esophagogastric anastomotic healing in the rat [47]. In an experiment involving 34 rats (two groups of 17), gastric tissue perfusion, measured in tissue perfusion units (TPU), decreased immediately after partial devascularization (before, 73.6±12.1 TPU;

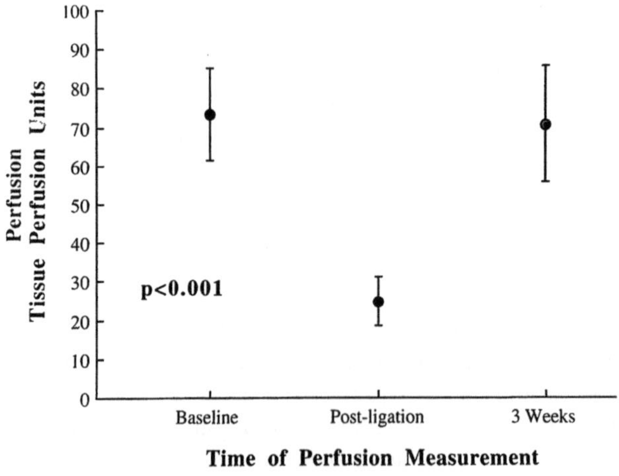

Fig. 1. Changes in rat gastric tissue perfusion after left gastric artery ligation, and a 3-week period of gastric ischemic conditioning [47]

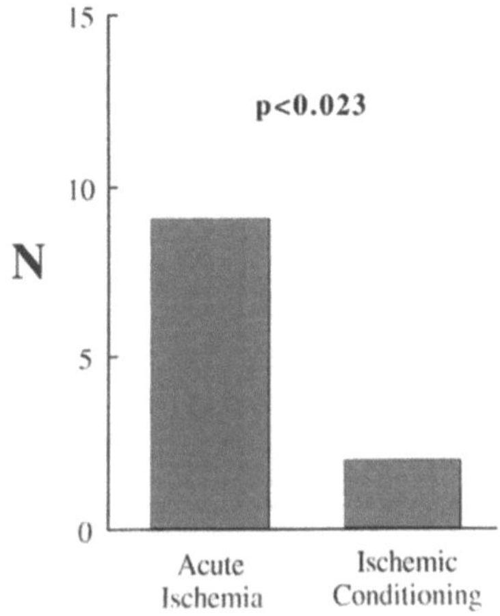

Fig. 2. Esophagogastric anastomotic dehiscence in rats with and without gastric ischemic conditioning [47]

after, 25.0±6.5 TPU; $p<0.001$). After 3 weeks, gastric tissue perfusion returned to baseline values in gastric-conditioned rats (before, 72.3±11.0 TPU; 3 week, 71.1±15.1 TPU; $p<0.80$) (Fig. 1). Gastric-conditioned rats had fewer anastomotic leaks (2 vs 9; $p<0.023$) and higher anastomotic wound-breaking strengths (2.35±1.05 N vs 1.56±0.76 N, $p<0.02$) than control rats (Fig. 2). Anastomotic wound hydroxyproline concentration was not significantly different in the two groups.

Gastric Conditioning: Clinical Applications

Clinical methods of gastric conditioning include two-stage esophagectomy (delayed anastomosis), preoperative gastric arterial embolization, and laparoscopic partial gastric devascularization. Two-stage esophagectomy and reconstruction is occasionally done in situations where anastomotic leakage is thought to be very likely. In this procedure, esophagectomy with or without gastric transposition is done at one operation, but creation of the anastomosis is delayed for 1–2 weeks (Fig. 3). During this time, gastric decompression is maintained with a retrograde jejunogastric tube, and the patient is nourished through a separate feeding jejunostomy tube [48]. Although experience with this two-stage procedure is limited, several investigators have noted a decrease in anastomotic leaks with its use [42, 49–52]. The benefits of the two-stage procedure have been attributed to the improved gastric vascularity that develops during the period of delay. These clinical observations are uncontrolled, but they support the hypothesis that gastric conditioning may reduce the incidence of esophagogastric anastomotic leaks.

Akiyama performed embolization of the left gastric, right gastric, and splenic arteries to improve gastric vascularity before esophagectomy [53]. After a 4-day to 38-day delay, esophagectomy was done and gastric-tube perfusion was measured by means of laser-Doppler flowmetry. In the emboliza-

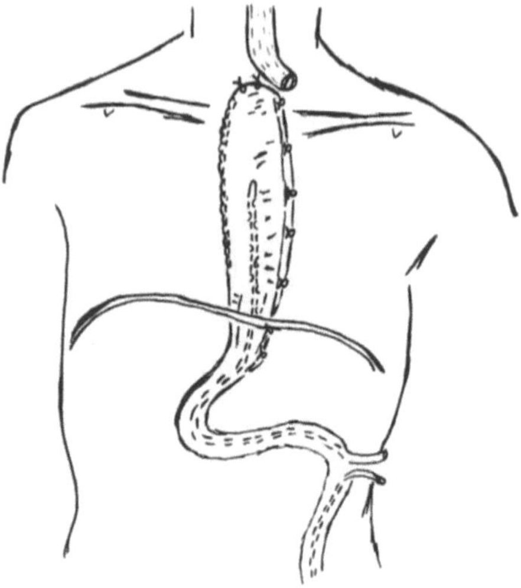

Fig. 3. Esophagectomy with delayed cervical esophagogastric anastomosis. Initially, the fundus is secured in the neck and an end esophagostomy is created. The anastomosis is done after a delay of 1–2 weeks

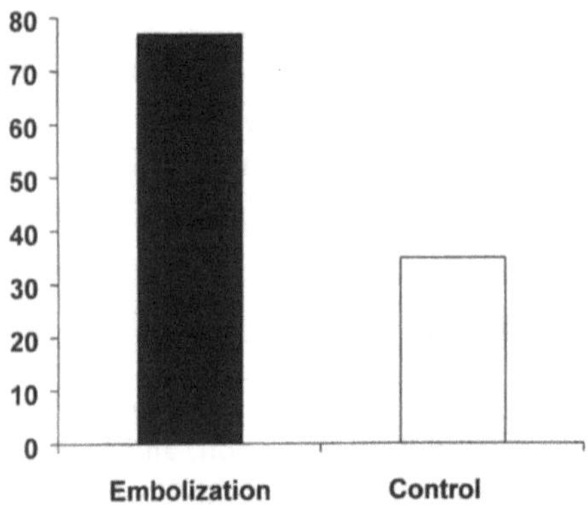

Fig. 4. Gastric-tube perfusion (expressed as a percentage of pre-mobilization gastric fundal perfusion) in patients treated with and without preoperative gastric arterial embolization [53]

tion group, gastric-tube perfusion was 77% of baseline values compared with 35% in a control group (Fig. 4). If embolization was done 8 days or more before esophagectomy, gastric-tube perfusion was 84% of baseline perfusion. When an arbitrary gastric-tube perfusion value of 50% of baseline was used as a criterion for acceptable gastric-tube vascularity, the embolization patients had significantly better perfusion than control patients (88% vs 8%, $p<0.001$) (Fig. 5). One minor anastomotic leak occurred in the 36 patients studied (embolization patient). Anastomotic leaks could not be predicted by intra-operative laser-Doppler flowmetry. Gastric conditioning by preoperative gastric-artery embolization could not be shown to reduce the incidence of esophagogastric anastomotic leaks.

Laparoscopic staging is useful for guiding cancer therapy; it has become a standard procedure in several esophageal cancer centers [54, 55]. Celiac and left gastric artery lymph nodes are exposed and sampled during laparoscopic

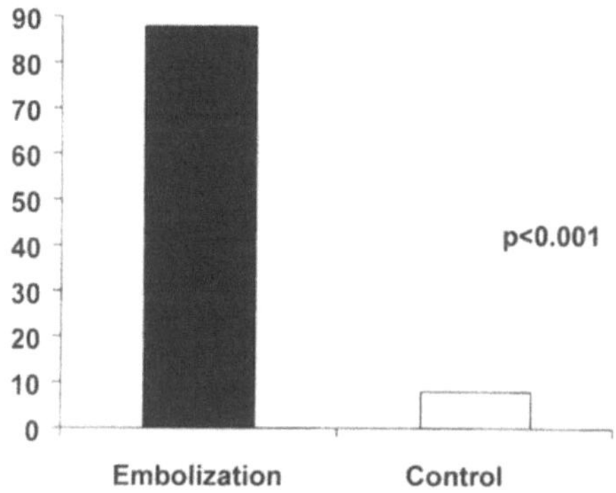

Fig. 5. Frequency of "acceptable" gastric-tube perfusion (>50% of baseline) in patients treated with and without preoperative gastric arterial embolization [53]

staging. Gastric conditioning can be accomplished by partial gastric devascularization at the time of laparoscopic staging [56]. The left gastric artery is ligated or clipped as lymph nodes in this region are dissected and sampled. To minimize possible hemorrhagic complications, the ligation is done in continuity (without vessel division). Other vessels, such as the short gastric arteries, may also be dissected and ligated, but this adds an additional risk of bleeding and splenic injury. Laparoscopic gastric conditioning at the time of laparoscopic staging is appealing, since gastric conditioning is achieved without requiring a separate procedure exclusively for the purposes of conditioning. Clinical pilot studies are underway.

Gastric Conditioning: Unanswered Questions

At this time, there is abundant evidence that gastric-tube blood supply can be improved by the process of gastric conditioning. However, insufficient gastric blood supply is not the sole cause of anastomotic leaks [2, 24]. Although there are data suggesting a reduction in anastomotic leaks with gastric conditioning, the evidence is far from conclusive. The extent of pre-esophagectomy partial devascularization required to condition the stomach is not known. Finally, overall treatment morbidity and cost of esophageal cancer treatment must be considered. Even if gastric conditioning reduces leaks, there is undoubtedly morbidity and cost associated with its use. For gastric conditioning to be clinically useful, the benefit from reduction in leaks must be greater than the costs and morbidity of the conditioning procedure itself.

References

1. Muller JM, Erasmi H, Stelzner M, Zieren U, Pichlmaier H (1990) Surgical therapy of oesophageal carcinoma. Br J Surg 77:845–857

2. Urschel JD (1995) Esophagogastrostomy anastomotic leaks complicating esophagectomy: a review. Am J Surg 169:634–640
3. Gelfand GAJ, Finley RJ, Nelems B, Inculet R, Evans KG, Fradet G (1992) Transhiatal esophagectomy for carcinoma of the esophagus and cardia: experience with 160 cases. Arch Surg 127:1164–1168
4. Tsui SL, Law S, Fok M et al (1997) Postoperative analgesia reduces mortality and morbidity after esophagectomy. Am J Surg 173:472–478
5. Schilling M, Redaelli C, Zbaren P et al (1997) First clinical experience with fundus rotation gastroplasty as a substitute for the esophagus. Br J Surg 84:126–128
6. Valverde A, Hay J-M, Fingerhut A, Elhadad A (1996) Manual versus mechanical esophagogastric anastomosis after resection for carcinoma: A controlled trial. Surgery 120:476–483
7. Bardini R, Asolati M, Ruol A, Bonavina L, Baseggio S, Peracchia A (1994) Anastomosis. World J Surg 18:373–378
8. Paterson IM, Wong J (1989) Anastomotic leakage: an avoidable complication of Lewis-Tanner oesophagectomy. Br J Surg 76:127–129
9. Law S, Fok M, Chu K-M, Wong J (1997) Comparison of hand-sewn and stapled esophagogastric anastomosis after esophageal resection for cancer: a prospective randomized controlled trial. Ann Surg 226:169–173
10. Beitler AL, Urschel JD (1998) Comparison of stapled and hand-sewn esophagogastric anastomoses. Am J Surg 175:337–340
11. Miller JD, Jain MK, de Gara CJ, Morgan D, Urschel JD (1997) The effect of surgical experience on results of esophagectomy for esophageal carcinoma. J Surg Oncol 65:20–21
12. Yamato T, Hamanaka Y, Hirata S, Sakai K (1979) Esophagoplasty with an autogenous tubed gastric flap. Am J Surg 137:597–602
13. Thomas DM, Langford RM, Russell RCG, Le Quesne LP (1979) The anatomical basis for gastric mobilization in total oesophagectomy. Br J Surg 66:230–233
14. Dei Poli M, Albertino B, Spalluto F et al (1990) Gastric angiography: data for oesophagogastroplasty. Panminerva Med 32:61–4
15. Liebermann-Meffert DMI, Meier R, Siewert JR (1992) Vascular anatomy of the gastric tube used for esophageal reconstruction. Ann Thorac Surg 54:1110–1115
16. Moorehead RJ, Wong J (1990) Gangrene in esophageal substitutes after resection and bypass procedures for carcinoma of the esophagus. Hepatogastroenterology 37:364–367
17. Miyoshi H (1986) Experimental and clinical studies on the viability of the stomach roll for esophageal reconstruction (in Japanese). Nippon Geka Gakkai Zasshi 87:499–509
18. Jacobi CA, Zieren HU, Muller JM, Adili F, Pichlmaier H (1996) Anastomotic tissue oxygen tension during esophagectomy in patients with esophageal carcinoma. Eur Surg Res 28:26–31
19. Abo S, Kitamura M, Hashimoto M et al (1996) Analysis of results of surgery performed over a 20-year period on 500 patients with cancer of the thoracic esophagus. Surg Today 26:77–82
20. Cooper GJ, Sherry KM, Thorpe JA (1995) Changes in gastric tissue oxygenation during mobilisation for oesophageal replacement. Eur J Cardiothor Surg 9:158–160
21. Salo JA, Perhoniemi VJ, Heikkinen LO, Verkkala KA, Jarvinen AA (1992) Pulse oximetry for assessment of gastric tube circulation in esophageal replacements. Am J Surg 163:446–447
22. Schilling MK, Redaelli C, Maurer C, Friess H, Buchler MW (1996) Gastric microcirculatory changes during gastric tube formation: assessment with laser doppler flowmetry. J Surg Res 62:125–129
23. Schilling MK, Mettler D, Redaelli C, Buchler MW (1997) Circulatory and anatomic differences among experimental gastric tubes as esophageal replacement. World J Surg 21:992–997
24. Pierie J-PEN, De Graaf PW, Poen H, van der Tweel I, Obertop H (1994) Impaired healing of cervical oesophagogastrostomies can be predicted by estimation of gastric serosal blood perfusion by laser doppler flowmetry. Eur J Surg 160:599–603

25. Sugimachi K, Ikeda M, Kai H, Ueo H, Okudaira Y, Inokuchi K (1982) Assessment of the blood flow in various gastric tubes for esophageal substitutes. J Surg Res 33:463-468
26. Machens A, Busch C, Bause Hw, Izbicki JR (1996) Gastric tonometry and drain amylase analysis in the detection of cervical oesophagogastric leakage. Br J Surg 83:1614-1615
27. Mannell A, Lambrechts H, Becker PJ, Oosthuizen MMJ (1990) The effect of acute blood loss and transfusion on the esophageal anastomosis. Res Surg 2:112-116
28. Kusano C, Baba M, Takao S et al (1997) Oxygen delivery as a factor in the development of fatal postoperative complications after oesophagectomy. Br J Surg 84:252-257
29. Dewar L, Gelfand G, Finley RJ, Evans K, Inculet R, Nelems B (1992) Factors affecting cervical anastomotic leak and stricture formation following esophagogastrectomy and gastric tube interposition. Am J Surg 163:484-489
30. Hermreck AS, Crawford DG (1976) The esophageal anastomotic leak. Am J Surg 132:794-798
31. Urschel JD (1993) Transplant delay will reduce anastomotic complications of gastric pull up for isolated esophageal atresia. Med Hypotheses 40:379-380
32. Ribuffo D, Muratori L, Antoniadou K et al (1997) A hemodynamic approach to clinical results in the TRAM flap after selective delay. Plast Reconstr Surg 99:1706-1714
33. Callegari PR, Taylor GI, Caddy CM, Minabe T (1992) An anatomic review of the delay phenomenon: I. Experimental studies. Plast Reconstr Surg 89:397-407
34. Taylor GI, Corlett RJ, Caddy CM, Zelt RG (1992) An anatomic review of the delay phenomenon: II. Clinical applications. Plast Reconstr Surg 89:408-418
35. Cederna PS, Chang P, Pittet-Cuenod BM, Razaboni RM, Cram AE (1997) The effect of the delay phenomenon on the vascularity of rabbit rectus abdominis muscles. Plast Reconstr Surg 99:194-205
36. Cederna PS, Chang P, Pittet-Cuenod BM, Razaboni RM, Cram AE (1997) The effect of the delay phenomenon on the vascularity of rabbit abdominal cutaneous island flaps. Plast Reconstr Surg 99:183-193
37. Reinisch JF (1974) The pathophysiology of skin flap circulation: The delay phenomenon. Plast Reconstr Surg 54:585-598
38. Cutting CB, Robson MC, Koss N (1978) Denervation supersensitivity and the delay phenomenon. Plast Reconstr Surg 61:881-887
39. Gottrup F, Oredsson S, Price DC, Mathes SJ, Hohn DC (1984) A comparative study of skin blood flow in musculocutaneous and random pattern flaps. J Surg Res 37:443-447
40. Jonsson K, Hunt TK, Brennan SS, Mathes SJ (1988) Tissue oxygen measurements in delayed skin flaps: a reconsideration of the mechanisms of the delay phenomenon. Plast Reconstr Surg 82:328-335
41. Williams DB, Payne WS (1982) Observations on esophageal blood supply. Mayo Clin Proc 57:448-453
42. Yannopoulus PA, Delis KT, Ioannides PG (1995) Subcutaneous transposition of the proximal oesophagus in oesophagoplasty: 8 years experience in 20 cases. Dis Esoph 8:53-56
43. Urschel JD (1995) Ischemic conditioning of the rat stomach: implications for esophageal replacement with stomach. J Cardiovasc Surg 36:191-193
44. Urschel JD (1996) The effect of ischaemia on anastomotic wound healing in the rat stomach. Med Sci Res 24:35-36
45. Urschel JD (1996) Ischaemic conditioning improves gastric wound healing in rats. Med Sci Res 24:307-308
46. Urschel JD, Takita H, Antkowiak JG (1997) The effect of ischemic conditioning on gastric wound healing in the rat: implications for esophageal replacement with stomach. J Cardiovasc Surg 38:535-538
47. Urschel JD, Antkowiak JG, DeLacure MD, Takita H (1997) Ischemic conditioning (delay phenomenon) improves esophagogastric anastomotic wound healing in the rat. J Surg Oncol 66:254-256

48. Urschel JD, Antkowiak JG, Anderson TM, Takita H (1998) Retrograde jejunogastric tube decompression after esophagectomy. J Surg Oncol 68:204–205
49. Sugimachi K, Inokuchi K, Natsuda Y, Kai H, Matsuura H (1983) Delayed anastomosis of the cervical portion of the esophagus in bypass operations for unresectable carcinoma of the esophagus. Surg Gynecol Obstet 157:233–236
50. Nabeya K (1995) Esophageal reconstruction: When to perform reconstruction. Dis Esoph 8:1–3
51. Lee Y, Fujita H, Yamana H, Kakegawa T (1994) Factors affecting leakage following esophageal anastomosis. Jpn J Surg 24:24–29
52. Gurski RR, Schirmer CC, Toneto JE Jr et al (1997) Delayed cervical anastomosis of the esophagus for esophageal carcinoma. Int Surg 82:56–59
53. Akiyama S, Ito S, Sekiguchi H et al (1996) Preoperative embolization of gastric arteries for esophageal cancer. Surgery 120:542–546
54. Bonavina L, Incarbone R, Lattuada E, Segalin A, Cesana B, Peracchia A (1997) Preoperative laparoscopy in management of patients with carcinoma of the esophagus and of the esophagogastric junction. J Surg Oncol 65:171–174
55. Stein HJ, Kraemer SJM, Feussner H, Fink U, Siewert JR (1997) Clinical value of diagnostic laparoscopy with laparoscopic ultrasound in patients with cancer of the esophagus or cardia. J Gastrointest Surg 1:167–173
56. Urschel JD (1997) Ischemic conditioning of the stomach may reduce the incidence of esophagogastric anastomotic leaks complicating esophagectomy: a hypothesis. Dis Esoph 10:217–219

Fundus Rotation Gastroplasty: A Modified Gastric Tube

M.K. Schilling, M.W. Büchler

Department for Visceral- and Transplantation Surgery, University of Bern, Inselspital, 3010 Bern, Switzerland

Abstract

Anastomotic failure remains to be one of the main problems in esophageal surgery with leakage rates up to 30% being reported currently. We addressed that problem by modifying the gastric-tube formation in utilizing all of the gastric fundus and omitting the resection of the lesser gastric curvature and accompanying vessels. Experimentally, those fundus-rotation gastroplasties were significantly longer and better perfused than conventional gastroplasties. In a clinical series of 53 patients (45 male, eight female, range 42–83 years) undergoing esophageal resection (49 malignancies, four non-malignant esophageal disease), four anastomotic leakages were found (7.5%). Three patients died due to a bronchial leak and adult respiratory distress syndrome, one with a complete gastric-tube necrosis and one with a colon perforation, sepsis and multiorgan failure. Eight patients developed a significant anastomotic stricture requiring repeated endoscopic dilatations. From our experimental and clinical experience, we conclude that the favorable length and perfusion of fundus-rotation gastroplasties allow for safe anastomosis at either the cervical or thoracic level.

Introduction

The stomach is the preferred and most physiological substitute for the esophagus. Two fundamentally different forms have been developed: isoperistaltic gastric tubes described by Jankowski without a resection of the lesser curvature and by Kirschner with resection of the lesser curvature or as anisoperistaltic tubes, first described by Jianu [1]. Both techniques were refined by Akiyama, Gavriliu, Beck and others [2–4]. One of the unsolved problems in esophageal substitution is anastomotic failure and its striking difference between occidental and oriental populations. Leakage rates up to 30% have been reported in the western literature [5, 6], but lower frequencies in the eastern literature [7, 8]. While some of those differences might be attributed to the diagnostic assessment and definitions of anastomotic leakage [9], they

Recent Results in Cancer Research, Vol. 155

might also be caused by anatomic differences in terms of stomach size [10] and anatomic variations of the blood supply of the greater curvature [11]. We addressed those anatomical variations by modifying the gastric-tube formation, utilizing all of the gastric fundus and omitting the resection of the lesser gastric curvature [12]. Experimentally, those fundus-rotation gastroplasties were significantly longer and better perfused than conventional gastroplasties [13] obtained by a complete resection of the lesser curvature, including resection of the blood supply along the lesser curvature.

In this article, we present the clinical results of the application of fundus-rotation gastroplasty in patients who underwent esophageal resection for malignant and benign esophageal disease.

Patients and Methods

Between November 1993 and November 1996, 92 patients were evaluated to undergo esophageal resection. Of these patients, 88 (94%) underwent an esophageal resection and 53 had the esophagus substituted by a fundus-rotation

Table 1. Demographic, oncological, and operative data of 53 patients undergoing esophagectomy and substitution of the esophagus by a fundus-rotation gastroplasty

Demographic data	
n	53
Male/female	45/8
Mean age	59(42–83) years
Weight loss	5.6±6 kg
ASA	3 (2–4)
Oncological data	
Squamous cell	37
Adeno	10
Others	2
Stage I	4
Stage II	10
Stage III	28
Stage IV	7
Operative data	
TTE	30
THE	23
Interposition	
Retrosternal	1
Mediastinal	
Anastomosis	
Pharyngeal	6
Cervical	37
Thoracic	10

ASA, risk score according to the American Society of Anesthesiology; *TTE*, transthoracic esophagectomy; *THE*, transhiatal esophagectomy.

gastroplasty. Those 53 patients were followed prospectively for the intra-operative, as well as their postoperative, course. Anastomotic leakage, defined as radiological leakage on a routine gastrografin swallow or clinical evidence for leakage and other surgical complications were the major evaluation criteria. ICU stay and total length of hospital stay were further evaluation criteria.

There were 45 male and eight female patients, with an average age of 59 years (range, 42–83 years). On admission, patients presented with an average weight loss of 5.6 kg (range, 0–30 kg); the mean anesthesiological risk score was 3. In all, 49 patients underwent esophageal resections for malignancies, including 37 patients with squamous cell carcinoma, ten patients with adenocarcinoma of the esophagus and two patients with other malignancies (one undifferentiated carcinoma, one undifferentiated sarcoma). Four patients underwent esophagectomy for other diseases. A thoracoabdominal esophagectomy was performed in 30 patients and the esophagus was resected transhiatally in 23 patients. A mediastinal route for the gastric tube was selected in 20 patients and a mediastinal route in 33 patients. The anastomosis was performed using a hand-sewn two-layer technique with an absorbable suture at the level of the pharynx in six patients, at the level of the cervical esophagus in 37 patients, and at the thoracic esophagus above the pulmonary veins in ten patients.

Technique of Fundus-Rotation Gastroplasty

After dissection of the greater and lesser curvature, the left gastric artery is severed at its truncal origin. A careful lymphadenectomy, including all connective tissue, is performed along the lesser curvature and the left gastric artery is resected at the lesser curvature. Frozen sections are obtained from those resected specimens. Fundus rotation gastroplasty is performed by stapling along the greater curvature with a distance of approximately 3 cm to the gastric border. Stapling is continued until sufficient length of the tube is obtained. Finally, the stapler line is inverted by interrupted sutures with a fine absorbable monofilament suture. Care has to be taken to preserve maximum length of the right gastric artery and the concomitant vein (Fig. 1) [12]. A pyloromyetomy is performed routinely.

Results

Fundus-rotation gastroplasty was performed in 53 patients. The average operative time was 7 h 20 min; time required for gastroplasty including lymphadenectomy ranges between 30 min and 45 min. A median of four red packed blood cells was transfused (range, 0–23).

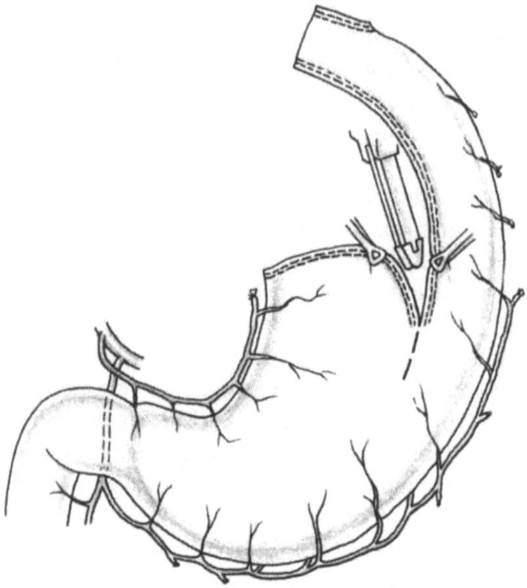

Fig. 1. Technique of fundus-rotation gastroplasty. After a careful lymphadenectomy along the lesser curvature, fundus-rotation gastroplasty is performed by stapling along the greater curvature with a distance of approximately 3 cm to the gastric border. The stapler line is inverted by interrupted sutures with a fine absorbable monofilament suture

Three of 53 patients died postoperatively, one as a result of a bronchial leak and adult respiratory distress syndrome, one of a complete gastric-tube necrosis, and one of a colon perforation, sepsis, and multiorgan failure.

A routine gastrografin swallow was performed between day 5 and day 7 postoperatively. In patients requiring prologed intubation, gastrografin swallow was performed after extubation. Four anastomotic leakages were found, three of these cervically. One thoracic anastomotic leak required re-operation with drainage and local irrigation. Further surgical complications included five laryngeal nerve pareses.

In total, 13 patients, including four with adult respiratory distress syndrome, suffered from pulmonary failure, requiring prolonged intubation. Eight patients required postoperative endoscopic dilatation of the esophagogastric anastomosis within 3 months postoperatively. A mean of five dilatations (range, 2–18) was required per patient.

Discussion

Anastomotic leakage after esophageal resection remains one of the major problems in esophageal surgery. It has prompted several studies that address technical aspects of the gastric substitute including the blood supply [14, 15]. These studies indicate that resection of the lesser curvature, as initiated

Table 2. Outcome in 53 patients undergoing esophagectomy and substitution of the esophagus by a fundus-rotation gastroplasty

Postoperative course	
Mortality[a]	3/53
Re-operation	3/53
Anastomotic failure	4/53
Length of hospital stay	24±13

[a] Inpatient mortality.

by Kirschner [16] and advocated by Akiyama and others, facilitates a radical resection of the draining lymphatic system, but also compromises the blood supply of the most peripheral segment of the gastric tube, the fundus remnant [15]. That remnant is solely supplied by the right gastroepiploic artery, which communicates with the left gastroepiploic artery in an extramural fashion only in one third of all patients [17]. We addressed this problem by maintaining the additional blood flow through the lesser curvature arcade and constructing a gastric tube from the gastric fundus only [12]. That tube was longer than conventional gastric tubes obtained through lesser curvature resection and better perfused than either conventional gastric tubes or reversed gastric tubes in an experimental model [13]. The application of fundus-rotation gastric tubes in a consecutive clinical series of 53 patients resulted in an overall leakage rate of 7.5%, irrespective of the level of anastomosis [18]. Even for high anastomosis at the pharyngeal level, there was ample gastric tube to perform a tension-free anastomosis and no anastomotic leakage was found in that subset of six patients. The grade of leakage was classified as minor and required a re-operation in one patient with a thoracic anastomosis. Anastomotic leakage in the series presented here was not associated with any further mortality; however, one patient with a complete stomach necrosis after neoadjuvant chemotherapy for squamous carcinoma of the esophagus died from subsequent sepsis. On revision laparotomy, the hiatus was found to be too narrow, thus compromising the blood supply in the gastroplasty in that patient. The favorable length and perfusion of fundus-rotation gastroplasties in both our experimental and clinical experience prompted us to additionally perform anastomosis at the thoracic level, depending only on oncological reasoning even in subgroups at high risk of anastomotic failure.

In view of the low anastomotic failure rate of fundus-rotation gastroplasty, however, one must not neglect oncological aspects such as the radicality and local recurrence after fundus-rotation gastroplasty with lymphadenectomy along the lesser curvature, which has to be addressed in further clinical prospective studies.

References

1. Lotheissen G (1922) Über plastischen Ersatz der Speiseröhre insbesondere aus dem Magen. Beitr Klin Chir 126:490–531
2. Akiyama H, Miyazono H, Tsurumaru M, Hashimoto C, Kawamura T (1978) Use of the stomach as an esophageal substitute. Ann Surg 188(5):606–610
3. Beck C, Carrel A (1905) Demonstration of specimens illustrating a method of formation of a prethora thic esophagus. Illi Med J 7:463–464
4. Gavriliu D, Georgescu L (1951) Esofagoplastie directacu material gastric. Rev Stiint Med 3:33–36
5. Bumm R, Hölscher AH, Fuessner H, Tachibana M, Bartels H, Siewert JR (1993) Endodissection of the thoracic esophagus. Technique and clinical results in transhiatal esophagectomy. Ann Surg 218(1):97–104
6. Borst HG, Dragojevic D, Stegmann T, Hetzer R (1978) Anastomotic leackage, stenosis and reflux after esophageal replacement. World J Surg 2:861–866
7. Akiyama H, Miyazono H, Tsurumaru M, Hashimoto C, Kawamura T (1978) Use of the stomach as an esophageal substitute. Ann Surg 188(5):606–610
8. Fok M, Chong AK, Cheng SWK, Wong J (1991) Comparison of a single layer continuous handsewn method and circular stapling in 580 esophageal anastomosis. Br J Surg 87:342–349
9. Bardini R, Asolati M, Ruol A, Bonavina L, Baseggio S, Peracchia A (1994) Anastomosis World J Surg 18:373–378
10. Goldsmith HS, Akiyama H (1979) A comparative study of Japanese and American gastric dimensions. Ann Surg 190(6):690–693
11. Koskas F, Gaiet B (1985) Anatomical study of retrosternal gastric esophagoplasties. Anat Clin 7:237–256
12. Büchler MW, Seiler Ch, Baer HU, Schilling MK (1996) A technique for gastroplasty as a substitute for the esophagus: fundus rotation gastroplasty. J Am Coll Surg 182:241–245
13. Schilling MK, Mettler D, Redaelli C, Büchler MW (1997) Differences between conventional, reversed and fundus rotation gastric tubes as esophageal replacement. World J Surg 21:1–5
14. Lindecken KD, Vogel J (1993) Die arterielle Durchblutung des Schlauchmagens beim Oesophagusersatz. Chir Gastroent 9:51–54
15. Liebermann-Meffert DMI, Meyer R, Siewert JR (1992) Vascular anatomy of the gastric tube used for esophageal reconstruction. Ann Thor Surg 54:1110–1115
16. Kirschner M (1920) Ein neues Verfahren der Oesophagusplastik. Arch Klin Chir 114:604–610
17. Yamato T, Hamanaka Y, Hirata S, Sakaj K (1979) Esophagogastroplasty with an autogenuous tubed gastric flap. Am J Surg 137:597–602
18. Schilling MK, Redaelli C, Zbären P, Baer HU, Seiler C, Friess H, Büchler MW (1997) First clinical experience with fundus rotation gastroplasty as a substitute for the oesophagus. Br J Surg 84:126–128

Colon Interposition

B. Cheng, K. Chen, S. Gao, Z. Tu

Department of Thoracic and Cardiovascular Surgery,
First Affiliated Hospital of Hubei Medical University, 430060 Wuhan, China

Abstract

In the anatomy of the colon vasculature, the ascending branch of the left colic artery is the primary supplying vessel (96.91%). Isoperistaltic transposition of the transverse colon is preferred (83.58%). Riolan's vascular arcade is not a major vessel of the colon. It can only be found in less than 10% of patients, and whether or not this arcade is complete cannot be used as criterion to judge colon blood supply. Animal experiments and clinical studies have confirmed the superiority of one-layer over two-layer anastomosis. The former is simpler, safer, and more reliable, with a lower incidence of anastomotic leak or stricture. Based on a comprehensive evaluation of the disease type, patient age, heart and lung functions, nutritional status, and accompanying diseases, three colon transposition routes are available (anterosternal subcutaneous tunnel, retrosternal tunnel, and esophageal bed passage). The advantages and disadvantages of each route are analyzed, and the left-middle-left retrosternal route is described. The indications for esophageal reconstruction with colon operation (ERC) were collected and verified, increasing the number of indications to seven categories of diseases. The main complications of ERC, i.e., colon segment necrosis, anastomotic leak, recurrent laryngeal nerve injury, and intestinal obstruction were systematically studied, and their causes and prevention are detailed. The number of patients is the highest in a single unit among all the published reports. The incidence of complications and deaths are the lowest.

Introduction

The stomach is the most commonly used substitute for esophageal reconstruction when the esophagus is resected because of diseases or loss of function. However, if there is a disease of the stomach or it has been resected, then the colon or jejunum is used as an alternative for reconstruction. With its adequate length, efficient blood supply, and high tolerance to irritations

Recent Results in Cancer Research, Vol. 155

by gastric juice, the colon is an ideal substitute for esophagus in total esophagectomy as it can avoid adverse effects on the respiratory and circulatory systems produced by pulling the stomach into the thoracic cavity. These advantages have already been well recognized [1–5]. However, the surgical procedure itself is very complex, involving many anastomoses, a risk of contamination and infection, and a high incidence of complications. If necrosis of the colon interposition occurs, the mortality rate is extremely high. These drawbacks have severely limited the application of this operation [1–5]. To address these problems, we carried out a series of studies on the structure and distribution of blood vessels in the colon, esophagocolonic anastomosis, selection of interposition routes, patterns of retrosternal routes, operation indications, and prevention and treatment of postoperative complications. As a result, for a total of 268 operation, our postoperative complication rate was reduced from 39% to 21.26%, and the mortality rate dropped to 2.23%.

Clinical Data

A total of 268 patients (193 male and 75 female), aged 2–72 years, underwent esophageal reconstruction with colon operation (ERC) between September 1962 and December 1996. The disease involved was esophageal cancer in 202 patients (75.37%), scar stricture of esophagus in 43 patients, spontaneous rupture of the esophagus in 13 patients, esophagotracheal fistula in five patients, multiple esophageal diverticula in one patient, reflux esophagitis with hemorrhage in two patients, and megaloesophagus in one patient. The colon segment interposition routes were via the anterosternal subcutaneous tunnel in 154 patients (57.46%), the retrosternal tunnel in 102 patients (38.05%), and the original esophageal bed in 12 patients: 160 patients 59.70% had curative esophageal resection, and 108 (40.3%) had esophageal bypass surgery only. Isoperistaltic positioning of the colon segment was performed in 224 patients (83.58%), and antiperistaltic positioning in 44 patients (16.42%). Pyloroplasty was simultaneously performed in 225 patients (83.95%).

Postoperative complications before discharge from hospital occurred in 57 patients (21.26%), and there were six deaths (2.23%). In early operations on 100 patients, the incidence of complications was 39%, which dropped to 10.71% in recent operations on 168 patients. In those patients in whom follow-up information was complete, the mean survival rate after esophageal cancer surgery ranged from 1 to 3 years; two of these patients survived 15 and 18 years, respectively, after curative surgery followed by radiotherapy and chemotherapy. One patient with late-stage esophageal cancer and concomitant hypertension, coronary heart disease, and pulmonary emphysema survived for 2 years after colon bypass. One patient with a malignant esophagotracheal fistula survived for 3 months after the bypass procedure. All the patients with benign esophageal diseases survived well and had normal lives and activities after 2–25 years of follow-up.

Colonic Vascular Structures and Patterns

A fatal complication that may occur after ERC is ischemic necrosis of the transpositioned colon segment. No such complication occurred in our series because the best supplying vessels were selected according to the conclusions drawn from research into colonic vascular distribution patterns and blood supply characteristics.

The starting points, cross ways, branching patterns, distributing areas, diameters, and blood supply of the middle, right, and left colonic arteries and their marginal vascular arcades were systematically observed and carefully recorded in the course of 162 operations [6]. The middle colic artery, which is the first branch of the superior mesenteric artery, lies in the midright segment of the transverse colon and supplies blood to one third to one half of the right part of the transverse colon. Its distributing areas are not constant, with 25.9% having no, two, or even more main stems. The branching patterns vary considerably, and 22.8% of the vessels have a V-shaped branch pattern or many parallel branches. The middle colic artery is therefore not the vessel of first choice for colon transposition. The right colic artery is the second branch of the superior mesenteric artery; it often branches out in a network fashion from the starting point. The vessels are weak and the marginal vascular arcade is not close enough to the colon. It is therefore even less suitable as a main supplying vessel for transplanted colon segment. We advocate the transposition of the transverse colon with the ascending branch of the left colic artery as the main supplying vessel for the following reasons: (a) the left colic artery is the first branch of the inferior mesenteric artery; (b) the ascending branch of this vessel is bulky, with a diameter similar to that of the middle colic artery; (c) it has a complete and consistent marginal vascular arcade, which does not spread in a network fashion; (d) the marginal vessels are very close to the colon at the splenic flexure, which is very suitable for stretching the colon; (e) the operative maneuver is easy; (f) most of the colon segment can be transpositioned isoperistaltically, which is physiologic. Based on these observations, we directly blocked the middle colic artery and the marginal vessels at the hepatic flexure at the beginning of operation and carefully observed the vascular arcade integrity at the splenic flexure and the vascular pulse status at the hepatic flexure of colon to be anastomosed to the esophageal stump. As a result of this innovation, the test time in which multiple vessels are blocked to find the ideal supplying vessels has been reduced from 25–30 min to 5 min. In recent years, we have performed 81 consecutive operations in which the transverse colon (with the left colic artery as its main supplying vessel) was transpositioned isoperistaltically. All were successful.

With respect to Riolan's vascular arcade in the colon, careful observations have found that it is not a major vascular arcade at the splenic flexure of the colon. Rather it is only a small tributary from the middle colic artery or the accessory middle colic artery. It runs into the retroperitoneal space. On the left side of the duodenojejunal flexure, it meets the accessory branch of the left colic artery and thus forms a vascular arcade. Only in less than 10% of patients can this vascular arcade be found, and whether or not this arcade is complete therefore cannot be regarded as a criterion to assess the colonic blood supply conditions [7].

Cervical Esophagocolostomy and Pharyngocolostomy

In our experiment with dogs, comparisons were made between one-row and two-row sutures. There was no anastomotic stenosis in either method. However, the fiber scar tissue was much thicker in two-row than in one-row sutures. Microscopic observations found no esophageal muscle twist, no gap formation at the suture line, and relatively less inflammatory cell infiltrations to the suture in one-row suture. This shows that two-row suture or sleeve suture requires mobilization of the esophagus up to 2.0–2.4 cm, while one-row suture only needs 1.0–1.2 cm of free esophagus. The latter can therefore ensure a more abundant blood supply to the anastomosis. In our series using one-row suture, the incidence of anastomotic leak decreases from 22.4% to 12.4% because of better blood flow to the anastomosis and slight inflammatory reactions [8–10].

In treating cervical esophageal cancer or chemical corrosion of the esophagus, the entire esophagus, including the starting portion, is often resected and replaced with colon. To ensure successful pharyngocolostomy, we adopted the following measures: (a) avoiding injury to the circular cartilage membrane when resecting the starting site of the esophagus; (b) avoiding injury to the superior laryngeal nerve and the recurrent laryngeal nerve when mobilizing the cervical esophagus; (c) using neat, interrupted sutures to secure the anterior, lateral, and posterior walls of the colon to the circular cartilage membrane, piriform recess mucosa, and the mucosa of the posterior wall of the pharynx, avoiding outward colonic mucosa; and (d) ensuring meticulous hemostasis to minimize infection. The loose tissues and abundant lymphoid tissue in the inferior pharyngeal region are prone to infection. A fine draining tube with many lateral openings is placed beneath the anastomosis [11].

Selection of Routes for Pulling Up the Colon Segment

Based on the clinical data and long-term follow-up, we believe that the subcutaneous anterosternal tunnel is suitable in elderly patients and patients with insufficient heart and lung function, a poor general condition, immune deficiency, diabetes mellitus, or an unresectable primary lesion. It can also be used in esophageal bypass surgery for cancer-induced esophagotracheal fistula. This route requires a relatively long colon segment for interposition [11]. The retrosternal tunnel is suitable in small children with scar stricture of the esophagus and in young patients with a long life-expectancy. These patients need good long-term functioning of both the esophagus and the stomach. As early as 1965, the present authors were the first to propose the left-right-left route pattern for retrosternal tunnel [12]. Along this route, the loose connective tissues at the level of the second and fourth rib cartilages were used close to the back of the sternum. The sternopericardial ligament was cut under direct visualization using a neck incision, and the tissue was separated along the back of the sternum. This method avoids rupture of pleura or injury to major blood vessels.

The posterior mediastinal esophageal bed passage is suitable for those patients whose stomach has already been partially resected, if total esophagectomy has to be performed because of serious gastric lesions, if a left neck incision has to be made, or if a combined left thoracoabdominal incision and a left neck incision are to be made. In this route, one-stage resection of the esophagus can be performed, and the colon segment is pulled up through the esophageal bed passage for neck anastomosis. In addition, this route is also suitable for segment resection of the diseases esophagus, in which the lower esophagus and gastric cardia are preserved and interpositioned colonically.

We also compared isoperistaltic and antiperistaltic ERC. In terms of esophageal physiology, the esophageal inlet is a high-pressure region. If an antiperistaltic ERC is performed, the antiperistalsis of the colon will increase the inner pressure at the anastomosis, which hinders healing. In our series, anastomotic leak occurred in 17 of 44 patients (36.63%) undergoing antiperistaltic ERC and in 11 of 224 patients (4.91%) undergoing isoperistaltic ERC ($p<0.01$). Thus we strongly advocate isoperistaltic ERC, not only because it is consistent with esophageal physiology, but also because it helps to reduce anastomotic leak [11, 13, 14].

Indications for Esophageal Reconstruction with Colon Operation

In 1911, Kelling and Vuliet were the first to describe ERC. Later, Rudler, Robertson, Battersky, Mononey, Mustart, and Scanlon reported their experience with ERC in treating congenital esophageal diseases and esophageal cancer. Our research began in September 1962, when ERC was performed to treat late-stage esophageal cancer. After that, we carried out a series of animal experiments and technical innovations. As a result, the incidence of complications and the mortality rate have dropped significantly, and the operation indications have gradually became broader. In our series, the ERC indications [9–12] are as follows:

- Scar stricture of the esophagus which fails to respond to repeated dilatation or other treatment. A 26-year-old woman underwent ERC after 108 painful dilatations in 5 years had failed to solve the problem. Following the operation, she regained her normal life and activities and gave birth to a healthy son (now 8 years old).

- Middle and upper esophageal cancer patients with previous gastrectomy or with gastric lesions.
- Extensive scar formation in the esophagus and stomach caused by chemical corrosion. In this case, reconstruction of the esophagus is required.
- Achalasia of the cardia which is not resolved by repeated operation, with severe reflux esophagitis leading to stricture.
- Long segment of spontaneous rupture of the esophagus.
- Multiple diverticula of the esophagus with perforation.
- Esophagotracheal fistula.
- Megaoesophagus.
- Esophageal atresia and segmental stenosis in infants [14].

Prevention and Treatment of Complications

The key to popularizing ERC lies in reducing the incidence of complications. Literature reports show that, although the overall incidence has decreased, it is still higher than that of esophageal replacement with stomach operation. Our research focused on the causes, effective prevention, and treatment of the following complications [11, 14].

Necrosis of the Colon Segment

Necrosis of the colon segment complication. In our series, we strictly selected and preserved the colonic vascular pedicle, maintaining the vascular arcade and preventing tension. No colon segement necrosis ever occurred. The measures taken to prevent this complication include the following:

1. Make sure that the supplying vessel to the colon is not obstructed and the mesocolon is not tense, not under pressure, and not twisted. If the left lobe of the liver is significantly enlarged, the mesocolon pedicle of the interposed colon should be pulled up through the gap between the left and the right lobes of the liver.
2. Avoid hypotension during operation.
3. Avoid pressing the cervical colon segment.

In early practice, a small piece of the manubrium of the sternum and sternoclavicular joints was routinely excised. Recent practice is to cut off all the tense connective tissues behind the manubrim at the thoracic outlet. Both procedures can achieve a satisfactory result.

Cervical Anastomotic Leak

Cervical anastomotic leak is a common nonfatal complication. However, if the leakage drains into the thoracic cavity or postmediastinum, the prognosis is poor. The causes are a poor general condition, local ischemia, serious contamination, and an inadequate surgical technique. However, a poor blood supply is a major cause. The preventive measures include the following:

1. Preserving good blood supply to the colon segment by choosing the ascending branch of the left colic artery.
2. Reducing the size of the large orifice of the transplant by suture on the opposite side of the mesocolon, making the cut margin on the mesocolon side 1 cm longer, and avoiding injury to the epiploic appendices of the colon.
3. Performing a single-layer esophagocolostomy with the correct tension and adequate space between the sutures. Care should be taken not to puncture blood vessels and not to leave any hematoma. When performing pharyngocolostomy, the anterior wall of the colon should be sutured inside-turned to the inferior pharynx.
4. Selecting a clear and unobstructed route to pull up the colon segment.
5. Isoperistaltic ERC is preferred.
6. Minimizing contamination of the operation field.
7. Avoiding severe coughing to prevent high-pressure air currents in the gastrocolonic cavity from hitting the anastomosis.

Recurrent Laryngeal Nerve Injury

If the nerve is pulled or stressed during operation, patients will suffer from temporary hoarse throat or dyspnea, and these symptoms will become permanent if the nerve is ligated or cut off. Preventive measures include the following:

1. Because the number of branches and location of branching are not constant and because of the complex relation of the nerve to fascia, we prefer not to free the whole nerve during the operation.
2. The nerve trunk runs along the tracheoesophageal groove adjacent to the trachea. Surgeons should push the outer layer of fiber tissue to the side of the trachea and avoid bulky ligation there.
3. Excessive pulling of the esophagus should be avoided to prevent injury to the nerve branches at the circular cartilage level.
4. Electric cutting or coagulation should be avoided in the deep neck and tracheoesophageal region.

Intestinal Obstruction

Intestinal obstruction is often related to the surgical procedure and often calls for reoperation. We had the following experience in early practice: (a) the colon segment was pulled up along the pregastric route, the mesocolon pressed on the stomach tightly, and dumbbell stomach occurred; (b) the colon segment was pinched by the rectal muscle sheath or the tight diaphragm; (c) the colon anastomosis was not in the dorsal region of the mesentery, which caused small-intestine obstruction; and (d) incomplete closure of the mesenteric incision led to intestinal hernia. Treatment involves reoperation to relieve obstruction and to repair and reconstruct the affected organs.

Cervical Anastomotic Stenosis

Cervical anastomotic stenosis is usually caused by scar tissues after the healing of anastomotic leak and local infection. It may also be caused by unduly early treatment for corrosive esophageal injury in which the scar tissue has not yet stabilized. Treatments include dilatation in the early stage, anastomotic plasty under local anesthesia for severe cases, or even resection of the stricture and reanastomosis.

Thoracic Colon Syndrome

Thoracic colon syndrome is similar to intrathoracic stomach syndrome. The symptoms include the inability to remain in a supine position, chest fullness, and being short of breath due to an enlarged colon after a meal. If the colon segment is placed subcutaneously, it is easy to see the peristalsis of the enlarged colon filled with air. The sound of peristalsis can also be heard. The causes are too big an anastomotic orifice, the anastomotic site being too close to the pylorus, a lengthy intra-abdominal colon segment causing angulation, or hypertrophic pylorus and stenosis of pylorus, making emptying difficult. Preventive measures include the following:

1. Cologastric anastomosis should be close to the cardia.
2. The orifice of anastomosis should be reduced in size to no more than 3 cm.
3. An antireflux technique should be adopted.
4. The inlet of the subcutaneous tunnel should be large enough, and the xiphoid and the erectus muscle should be excised along with its anterior and posterior sheath to make a hole 3 cm in diameter.
5. The colon segment should be interposed isoperistaltically.

Esophageal Pouch Syndrome

Esophageal pouch syndrome is a syndrome of sustained substenal and dull back pain produced by the accumulation of mucus in the leftover esophagus. X-ray examination and ultrasonography reveal a large cyst in the end-to-side anastomosis in the leftover esophagus. Preventive measures include the following:

1. Avoiding the end-to-side anastomosis.
2. Using one-stage resection of the esophagus.

3. If the esophagus has to be left over, before closing the resection end, the contents of the esophageal cavity must be thoroughly drained, the cavity washed, and the mucosa completely destroyed by chemical corrosion. This can promote scar formation to close the stump. Another method is to insert a fine tube into the pouch and to inject sclerosing agents regularly until the pouch closes.
4. Managing to resect the esophageal pouch.

Conclusion

As a result of our result, we have achieved a wider clinical application, a large number of patients, a low complication rate, and a low mortality rate. Among the reports in the literature, both foreign and domestic, we have had the largest number of patients in a single unit (286), the lowest complication rate (21.26%), and the lowest mortality rate (2.23%).

The indications have been extended to cover seven categories of disease, with malignant lesions accounting for 77.23% and benign lesions for 22.77%. The surgical methods used are (a) total esophagectomy with esophageal reconstruction using colon, (b) esophageal bypass using colon to replace esophagus, with the diseased esophagus left over, and (c) partial esophagectomy with colon interposition to restore esophageal continuity.

References

1. Coleman JJ III (1995) Reconstruction of the pharynx and cervical esophagus. Semin Surg Oncol 11:208–220
2. Peters JH, Kronson JW, Katz M et al (1995) Arterial anatomic considerations in colon interposition for esophageal replacement. Arch Surg 130:858–862
3. Cerfolio RJ, Allen MS, Deschamps C et al (1995) Esophageal replacement by colon interposition. Ann Thorac Surg 59:1382–1384
4. Urschel JD (1996) Late dysphagia after presternal colon interposition. Dysphagia 11:75–77
5. Ahmad SA, Syivester KG, Hebra A (1996) et al Esophageal replacement using the colon: is it a good choice. J Pediatr Surg
6. Cheng BC, Gao SZ, Tu ZF et al (1989) Clinical observation of colic vessels with respect to their significance in the replacement of the esophagus by colon. Chin J Surg 27:566–568
7. Cheng BC, Gao SZ (1995) Anatomical study on the Riolan's anastomosis arch. Chin J Surg 33:232–233
8. Gao SZ, Wang TS, Yao Z et al (1988) Experimental study and clinical application of a single row suturing esophagogastrostomy. Chin J Surg 26:665–666
9. Gao SZ, Cheng BC, Tu ZF et al (1990) Experimental study and clinical application of a single-row suturing esophagogastrostomy. J Surg Oncol 42:167–170
10. Gao SZ, Cheng BC, Tu ZF et al (1992) Experimentelle Untersuchung und klinische Anwendung der esophagealen einreihigen Allschichtennahtanastomose. Chir Gastrienterol 8:372–375
11. Tu ZF, Gao SZ, Yao Z (1987) The improved technique of colon interposition. Chin J Thorac Cardiovasc Surg 3:95–96

12. Gao SZ (1965) The technique for retrosternal tunnel. Chin J Surg 3:680–682
13. Cheng BC, Lin DM, Tu ZF et al (1994) Colon replacement of esophagus: clinical experience of 252 cases. Chin J Thorac Cardiovasc Surg 10:236
14. Cheng BC, Gao SZ, Tu ZF t al (1997) Management complications in colon replacement for esophagus. Chin J Thorac Cardiovasc Surg 1391–1393

Complications Following Esophageal Surgery

Ö. P. Horváth, L. Lukács, L. Cseke

First Department of Surgery, University Medical School of Pécs, Ifjusag U. 13., 7643. Pécs, Hungary

Abstract

Chronologically, complications can be classified as intraoperative, early, and late. The authors analyze complications according to this classification on the basis of more than 400 esophageal operations and related literary data. As regards intraoperative complications, they deal only with those occurring at transhiatal esophagectomy (e.g., tracheal tear, bleeding, pneumothorax, laryngeal nerve injury). Among the early complications, they survey the incidence of transplant necrosis and related mortality, further sequelae ensuing from subacute ischemia of the replaced organ and analyze in detail the questions which arise regarding anastomotic leakage. Firstly, they deal with those causative factors that influence the frequency of anastomotic insufficiency, such as the technical "know-how" of anastomosis making (e.g., one layer vs two layers; stapling or manual suture; interrupted or running suture), the way of replacement using whole stomach or tube-stomach and the consequences originating from the route of replacement (e.g., anterior or posterior mediastinal route). Incidence and management of chylothorax are also dealt with.

While dealing with late complications, the authors give a detailed comment on anastomotic strictures and also other factors facilitating the development of late dysphagia, such as peptic stricture and tumor of the organ remnant.

Finally, some cases successfully treated by surgery are presented (skin-tube formation in cases following transplant necrosis; abolition of a pharyngogastric anastomosis stricture using a free jejunal transplant and surgical solution of an anastomotic stricture from median sternotomy approach).

Introduction

A complication can be regarded as an event arising either during the course of the intervention or during the postoperative phase that may alter the course of intervention or its usual length of time. Furthermore, it may extend the term of intensive postoperative care and/or hospital stay and neces-

Recent Results in Cancer Research, Vol. 155

sitate therapeutic interventions other than routine interventions. Due to these factors, the cost of treatment will be increased.

The notion of complication is unclearly defined and, therefore, it seems rather unwise to create a total number of complications. However, it is more expedient to emphasize the leading complications and to compare them according to the type of operation and the different operative institutions. Chronologically, complications can be classified as intraoperative, early, and late. The latter includes complications occurring after 30 days.

In this chapter, while trying to touch on all possibilities involved, I would like primarily to discuss anastomotic insufficiency and the so-called late complications of esophageal surgery in detail. As a matter of fact, it is not worth mentioning intraoperative complications, except in cases of transhiatal esophageal resection and complications arising thereof which may indeed alter the course of the operation (e.g., one should proceed with thoracotomy), or influence the postoperative period (e.g., with ptx), and where recurrent nerve palsy and/or pulmonary complications are more frequent.

Bleeding and tracheal injury necessitating thoracotomy total 1% in institutions with great expertise (Table 1). In cases of tracheal injury, it is highly justifiable to perform esophageal replacement in the posterior mediastinum as the gastric wall can be sutured onto the injury site as a cover-patch. In one of our three cases, the tracheal lesion was caused, without any doubt, by the tracheal tube that disrupted the pars membranacea, in a thin female weighing less than 40 kg, after the esophagus behind it had been removed. The suture of the trachea was covered in one case by a pericardium patch, and in two cases with gastric wall. Two patients recovered.

The opening of the mediastinal pleura is deemed in itself a harmless event, though we demonstrated that pulmonary complications, as well as anastomotic dehiscence, occurred more frequently in these cases. The latter may be caused by hypoxia due to impaired pulmonary function, but stretching of the anastomosis may also play a role, whereby the stomach does not remain in the midline, but slides easily through the opened pleura into one of the thoracic cavities. The frequency of recurrent palsy at three-field lymphadenectomies may also reach 50% [10].

Table 1. Intraoperative complications during transhiatal esophagectomy

Reference	Number	Tracheal tear (%)	Bleeding (%)	Pneumothorax (%)	Laryngeal nerve injury (%)
Moreno-Gonzales et al. 1992 [20]	281	0.6	0.3	–	–
Orringer et al. 1993 [22]	583	0.6	0.5	74	3
Geemo 1985 [23]	838	1.5	8.6	13.2	23.2
Katariya et al. 1994 [16]	1353	0.7	1.3	–	11.3
Peracchia et al. 1992 [25]	140	1.5	0.7	–	10
Horváth 1997 [14]	115	2.6	0.9	41	15

Table 2. Necrosis of the substitute

Reference	Number	Necrosis (%)	Successful reconstruction	Uncompleted reconstruction
Moorehead and Wong 1990 [19]				
Stomach	416	1.2	–	–
Colon	44	13.6	–	–
Peracchia et al. 1992 [24]				
Stomach	95	10.5	2	–
Colon	11	18	–	2
Altorki et al. 1994 [2]				
Stomach	75	4	1	2
Hanaoka et al. 1995 [11]				
Stomach	306	2.3	1	–
Colon	32	9.4	2	–
Collard 1997 [7]				
Stomach	257	1.5	1	–
Horváth 1997 [14]				
Stomach	310	2	2	1
Colon	50	8	1	–

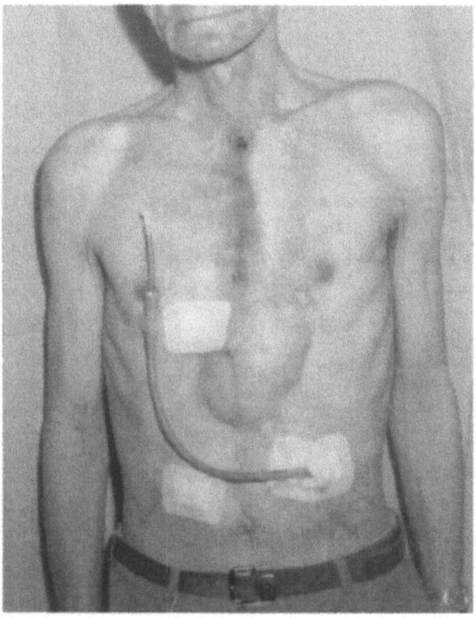

Fig. 1. Patients who survived two instances of transplant necrosis; the final reconstruction was achieved with a skin tube made from musculo-cutaneous flaps

Of the possible early complications, necrosis of the replaced organ is the most dangererous and is associated with the highest mortality rate. According to literary data (Table 2), necrosis of the gastric tube is less frequent (about 1%–2%), while necrosis of the colon stands at 10%. Peracchia's data, shown in Table 2, refer to the treatment of tumors of the cervical esophagus, thus the high rates [24]. Necrosis of the replaced organ leads in 90% of cases to a fatality. Reconstruction is only successful in barely more than one half of the survivors, and the rest of the patients remain on tube feeding through

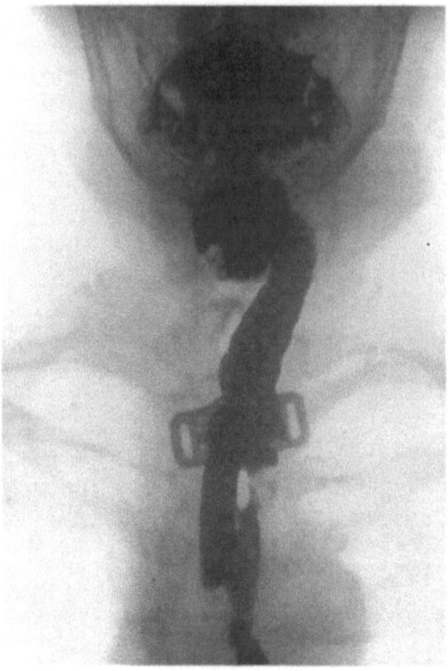

Fig. 2. Subacute ischemic signs in a free jejunal transplant. Mucosal contour disappeared

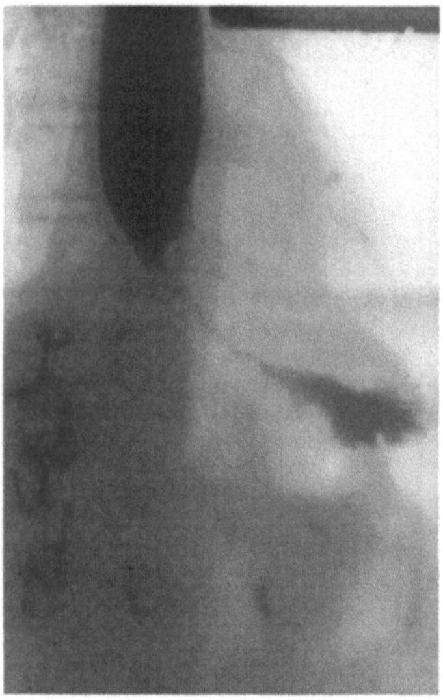

Fig. 3. Long ischemic stricture in a Roux-loop used for esophagoplasty

a gastrostomy for life. In one case, following a substernal gastric replacement, we were forced to perform a presternal colonic replacement. After this procedure, the upper third of the colon necrotized. This was resected and, in a subsequent setting, a neo-esophagus was created using musculo-cutaneous flaps. The patient is in a satisfactory condition and, at present, a survivor of 2 years. The first layer was made by means of a so-called reverse pectoral flap. The ensuing defect was covered by a musculo-cutaneous flap taken from

Table 3. Prognostic factors for esophageal anastomotic leakage

Anatomic
Lack of serosa, fragile muscle layer, impaired blood supply
Nutritional status
Co-morbid states
Metabolic, hepatic, cardiac respiratory disorders
Tumor related
Tumor stage
Bypass or resection
Cancer at resection margin
Tension of anastomosis
Blood supply of the substitute
Suture material
Kind of anastomosis
Mechanical or manual
One layer or two layers
Interrupted or running suture
Level of the anastomosis
Gastric emptying
Route of reconstruction
Gastric tube or whole stomach
Postoperative complications
Surgeon's experience (!!)

the latissimus dorsi muscle. In Fig. 1, the patient is shown 3 months after reconstruction.

Subacute ischemia represents a complication that is infrequently observed and only occasionally discussed. The disturbed blood supply generally does not impair anastomotic healing, but may have late consequences. Inexplicable fever in the patient and discharge of mucosal debris through the nasogastric tube laid for decompression may comprise the clinical symptoms. Radiological signs include: thumb printing on the mucosal contour, irregular and flattened mucosal villi, mucosal denudation, and segmental stenosis.

In Fig. 2, mucosal denudation is visible in a free jejunal transplant, which, on this occasion, proved to be reversible, while in Fig. 3, a long, segmental stricture of the Roux-limb is shown, having been used for esophageal replacement.

Esophageal anastomosis is still associated with a high rate of complications, even though this has decreased considerably in recent years. Prognostic factors are summarized in Table 3.

As with wound healing, anastomotic healing is also influenced by local and systemic factors. Considering the anatomy of the esophagus, the lack of a serosal coat is significant, but it has a stronger mucosa and submucosa. "Impaired" blood supply is probably not a factor, because segments of 5–6 cm or longer can be isolated without evidence of ischemia and, if a re-operation is carried out due to anastomotic dehiscence, the esophagus is never ischemic and therefore is not responsible for the complication.

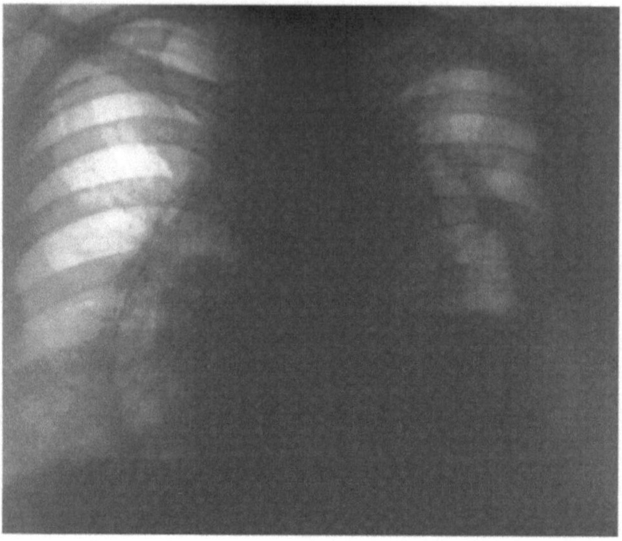

Fig. 4. The whole stomach can greatly expand during the early postoperative period, despite permanent nasogastric decompression

Multiple systemic factors influence healing of the anastomosis: malnutrition, hypoxia, hypovolemia, uremia, jaundice, diabetes mellitus, chemotherapy, and advanced age. There is controversy surrounding whether or not tumor stage and histologically positive resection margin influence anastomotic healing. The rate of anastomotic leakage, on the basis of the cited references, is significantly higher following bypass operations than after esophageal resection [14].

A suture line void of stretching is thought to be a basic requirement for anastomoses. At intramediastinal replacement following transhiatal esophagectomy, it may happen that the gastric tube of an appropriate length will slip into one of the thoracic cavities due to the lesion in the mediastinal pleura, an event that may put the anastomosis under strain.

Adequate perfusion and oxygenation are critical requirements for anastomotic healing. Ishigami and Kudo [15, 17] were able to demonstrate that both the thoracal sympathectomy and thoracal epidural anesthesia improved blood circulation of the gastric transplant. I can also confirm this statement on the basis of my own favorable experience.

Dilatation of the stomach pulled up into the thorax will result as a rule in deteriorated intramural circulation. Dilatation of the stomach may come about even with synchronous nasogastric tubing and the distended stomach can be the source of further, cardiorespiratory problems. This is the well-known argument against a total gastric transplant (Fig. 4).

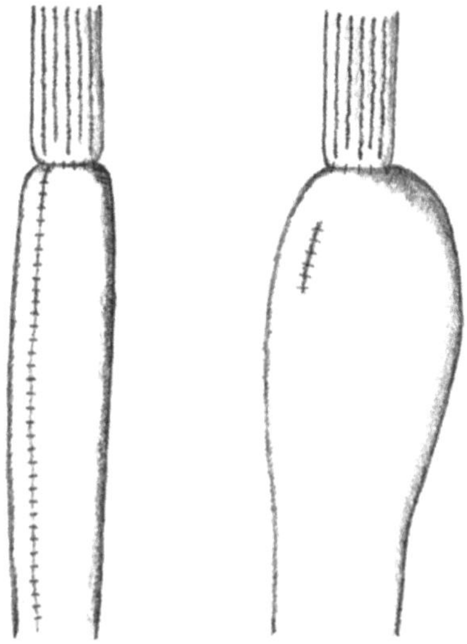

Fig. 5. Esophago-gastric anastomosis with a gastric tube (*left*) and with a whole stomach (*right*). The meeting point of the two suture lines of the gastric tube predisposes to ischemia

Table 4. Gastric tube or whole stomach leakage rate

Whole stomach, large gastric tube		Narrow gastric tube	
Author	Leakage rate (%)	Author	Leakage rate (%)
Bardini [4]	4.8	Fekete [9]	16
Lam [18]	4.7	Ribet [27]	23.3
Orringer [22]	8	Zieren [30]	11
Akiyama [1]	1.3	Pierie [26]	15
Collard [7]	1.4	Collard [7]	7.3
Average	4	Average	14.7

However, there are some arguments in favor of a total gastric transplant:

- Collard [7] showed that blood from the right gastroepiploic artery will get through the intramural capillary network adjacent to the lesser curvature to the site of the anastomosis, i.e., the fundus.
- Performance of an esophago-gastric anastomosis is greatly facilitated in the whole stomach by the fact that the cardiac staple line is located distal of the anastomotic site in the fundus, while, in the case of a gastric tube, the existence of a T-suture line is a weak point of the anastomosis (Fig. 5).

According to an overview of the literary data (Table 4), the rate of anastomotic dehiscence following the use of a total gastric transplant was found to be 4%, while after operations using a narrowed gastric tube for replacement, this rate was approximately 14.7%. The difference is significant.

The number of anastomotic complications does not depend on the quality of the suturing material. There is an observable trend to use ever thinner thread for suturing esophageal anastomoses. According to the literary data

Table 5. Anastomotic leakage rate with interrupted or running suture (own material)

	Interrupted (1986–1992)	Running suture (1992–1997)
Stomach	88 (18) 20.4%	124 (15) 12%
Jejunum [a]	42 (2) 4.7%	44 (1) 2.2%
Colon	19 (3) 15.8%	31 (4) 12.9%

[a] Cardia tumors are included.

Table 6. Reconstruction in the anterior or posterior mediastinum

Advantages of posterior mediastinal route
Shorter length of the route
Gastric motility more physiologic (deglutive function is better)
No need for a second tunnel
The diameter of the thoracic inlet is wider posteriorly than anteriorly
The stomach can protect the tracheo-bronchial tree
Dilatation is easier
Less respiratory complications
Leakage rate is lower (?)
Advantages of anterior mediastinal route
Leakage has less serious consequences (?)
Re-operation is easier
Postoperative radiotherapy is possible
Recurrent tumor in mediastinum does not cause dysphagia

[3], there is no significant difference between manual and mechanical anastomoses; however, high thoracic anastomoses are better sutured using a stapler, while the cervical anastomoses manually.

Prospective, randomized studies have proven that there is no significant difference between one-layer and two-layer anastomoses with respect to the incidence of early postoperative complications [30].

In accordance with the former statement, numerous authors found no difference between the results of one-layer knotted and one-layer running sutures [4]. According to our experience, both early and late results of a running suture are better than those after knotted sutures (Table 5). Hermetic and watertight sutures are easier to achieve using a running suture and also preferable in order to prevent anastomotic dehiscence. In my opinion, running sutures are more advantageous for cervical anastomoses, because, in the neck, at the level of the anastomosis, the intraluminal pressure is higher than in the lower segment of the esophagus, thus the watertight condition is of greater importance.

The necessity of an additional pyloroplasty is also debated. Some studies reported an increased rate of anastomotic complications without pyloroplasty; the majority of authors, however, did not find any significant difference [3, 31]. As for myself, I always perform a pyloroplasty. In two cases, on returning home from a congress, I tried to omit pyloroplasty, but the complications which appeared soon thereafter made me go back to my former practice.

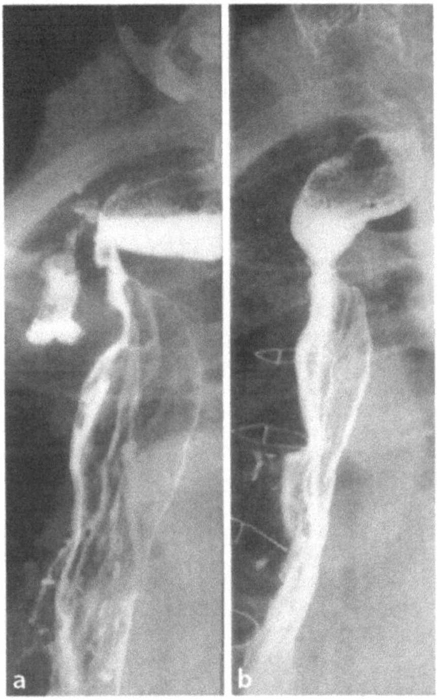

Fig. 6. a Esophago-gastric anastomosis insufficiency after anterior mediastinal replacement. A significant angulation can be seen at the level of the anastomosis. **b** Re-operation was performed from a median sternotomy approach, and, thereafter, the angulation disappeared and swallowing was normal

An important factor influencing the establishment of anastomotic leakage is the mode of reconstruction. From the point of view of possible anastomotic dehiscence, the posterior mediastinal route seems to be more favorable since the pull-up here is the shortest, the thoracic inlet is wider posteriorly than anteriorly, and there is no kinking between the axis of the gullet and the stomach [5]. Further advantages of the posterior route are detailed in Table 6.

Between the axis of the stomach pulled up anteriorly and that of the esophagus, there is often a conspicuous kinking, and this angulation is not infrequently at the level of the anastomosis (Fig. 6a). However, the anterior route also has its own advantages - precisely as a result of the kinking and pressure conditions, dehiscence arises mostly on the anterior wall and its consequences are therefore milder. Occasional dilatation due to the kinking can be more difficult; although, at the same time, re-operation, if the need arises, is relatively easy to perform using a median sternotomy approach.

The leak incidence after both mechanical and manual anastomoses is much higher in collective reviews than in reports from leading centers. "Frequent" esophageal surgeons can learn from their previous experience and therefore avoid technical errors, whereas "casual" surgeons do not have this opportunity [4].

The most frequent complication of esophageal surgery is related to the respiratory system. Indeed, this topic merits a chapter of its own, and thus I

Table 7. Frequency of chylothorax as a complication of esophagectomy

Reference	Number	Chylothorax (%)
Orringer et al. (1988) [21]	320	3
Siewert et al. (1988) [28]	121	1.6
Bolger (1991) [6]	537	2.0
Dougenis (1992) [8]	255	3.9
Horváth (1997) [14]	360	0.83

Table 8. Prevalence of cervical anastomotic stricture

Author	Stricture (%)
Bardini (1994) [4]	9.5
Orringer (1993) [22]	10
Lam (1992) [18]	7.7
Wang (1992) [29]	25.1
Zieren (1993) [30]	
Double layered	48
Single layered	19
Horváth (1997) [14]	
Interrupted suture	24
Running suture	8

do not intend to go into details now. One point, however, should be stressed here: In the case of a respiratory complication, it is always important to first exclude surgical complication or failure, since these very often constitute the underlying problem. However, at the same time, respiratory complications with associated hypoxia and repeated deglutition of infected sputum may inversely also lead to surgical complications.

Chylothorax represents a special complication of thoracic surgery, with an incidence rate of 1%–3% in large groups of patients (Table 7). It is generally accepted that the best results are obtained by early surgical intervention. Three of our patients underwent re-operation for this complication within 7 days, and all recovered.

Dysphagia is perhaps the most frequent late complication of esophageal replacement. Among its causes, anastomotic stricture is the most important and most frequent finding. According to literary data, anastomotic strictures occur in 3%–50% (Table 8), and possibly more often following mechanical anastomosis, particularly if small magazines have been used. Dehiscences healing spontaneously are, as a rule, followed by an anastomotic stricture at a rate of 50%–70%. The suturing technique also represents an influencing factor. In Zieren's study [30], it occurred more frequently after two-layer anastomoses, while, on the other hand, we had a favorable experience when using the running suture technique, even for late strictures.

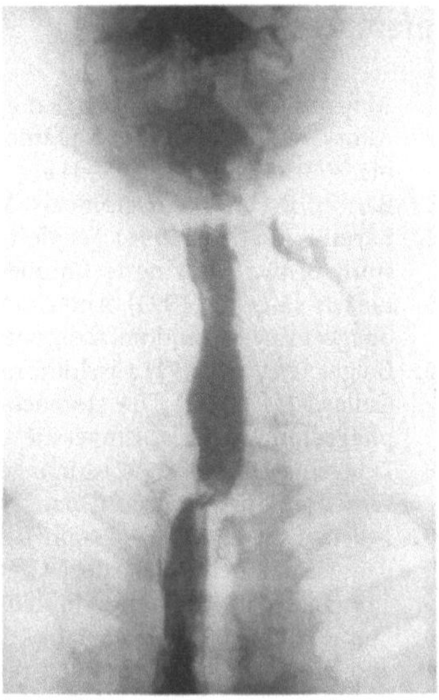

Fig. 7. Due to an undilatable pharyngo-gastric anastomotic stricture, a free jejunal graft interposition was performed

The first choice of treatment for anastomotic strictures should be dilatation. Dilatative treatment, however, is difficult if there is a significant angulation at the level of the anastomosis, such as after substernal replacement. In such cases, one should decide to proceed with re-operation. We have performed successful re-operation on five patients using the median sternotomy approach (Fig. 6b). There was no need for re-operation among patients treated with posterior mediastinal replacement.

Pharyngo-gastric anastomoses are also prone to develop strictures. In one of our patients, anastomotic stricture occurred after spontaneous healing of a dehiscence. We were not able to dilate successfully and solved the situation by using a free jejunal-loop transplant (Fig. 7).

Ischemic strictures are rare complications and usually occur after jejunal or colonic replacement. Short strictures can be treated with dilatation, but long segment strictures should generally be re-operated. Peptic strictures are mostly seen after thoracal esophago-gastrostomy.

Tumors may develop after esophageal resection in the esophagus remnant. In one of our patients, an adenocarcinoma was found in the esophagus remnant 18 years after the resection of a peptic esophageal stricture and jejunal transplant, probably due to Barrett's metaplasia of the post-resectional segment [13]. Furthermore, a tumor may also develop in the organ used for replacement, for example in a skin tube - as we experienced - which had been constructed 46 years earlier. The skin tube was removed and, subsequently, an antethoracal colonic replacement was performed while the defect was covered by a musculo-cutaneous flap taken from the latissimus dorsi muscle [14].

References

1. Akiyama H (1973) Esophageal anastomosis. Arch Surg 107:512–514
2. Altorki NK et al (1994) Squamous cell carcinoma of the esophagus: therapeutic dilemma. World J Surg 18:308–311
3. Bardini R (1994) Anastomosis. World J Surg 18:373–378
4. Bardini R et al (1994) Single-layered cervical esophageal anastomoses: a prospective study of two suturing techniques. Ann Thorac Surg 58:1089–1090
5. Bartels H et al (1993) Anterior versus posterior reconstruction after transhiatal oesophagectomy: a randomized controlled trial. Br J Surg 80:1141–1144
6. Bolger C et al (1991) Chylothorax after oesophagectomy. Br J Surg 78:587–588
7. Collard JM (1997) The stomach as an esophageal substitute after total or subtotal esophagectomy. Thesis, Université Catholique de Louvain
8. Dougenis D et al (1992) Management of chylothorax complicating extensive esophageal resection. Surg Gynecol Obstet 174:501–506
9. Fekete F et al (1988) Prophylactic operative techniques: 380 esophageal anastomoses using stapler. In: Delarue NC et al (eds) Esophageal cancer. Mosby, St Louis, pp 119–129 (International trends in general thoracic surgery, vol 4)
10. Fujita H et al (1995) Mortality and morbidity rates, postoperative course, quality of life and prognosis after extended radical lymphadenectomy for esophageal cancer: comparison of three-field lymphadenectomy with two-field lymphadenectomy. Ann Surg 222:654–662
11. Hanaoka T et al (1996) Necrosis in esophagus reconstruction organs after esophageal cancer resection. In: Peracchia A et al (eds) Diseases of the esophagus. Manduzzi Editore, Bologna, pp 267–271
12. Horváth ÖP et al (1991) Skin cancer: a late complication of skin tube oesophagus. Br J Surg 78:1467–1468
13. Horváth ÖP et al (1993) Adenocarcinoma arising in Barrett's esophagus after esophageal resection and jejunal interposition. In: Nabeya K et al (eds) Diseases of the esophagus. Springer, Berlin Heidelberg New York, pp 150–155
14. Horváth ÖP, Lukács L (1996) Palliation of esophageal cancer: palliative resection and bypass surgery. Dis Esoph 9:117–122
15. Ishigami K et al (1988) Neurovascular manipulation for safer surgery of thoracic esophageal cancer. In: Siewert JR, Hölscher AH (eds) Diseases of the esophagus. Springer, Berlin Heidelberg New York, pp 437–442
16. Katariya K et al (1994) Complications of transhiatal esophagectomy. J Surg Oncol 57:157–163
17. Kudo et al (1988) Prognosis of esophageal substitute in tissue viability and anastomotic leakage. In: Siewert JR, Hölscher AH (eds) Diseases of the esophagus. Springer, Berlin Heidelberg New York, pp 522–525
18. Lam TFC et al (1992) Anastomotic complications after esophagectomy for cancer. A comparison of neck and chest anastomosis. J Thorac Cardiovasc Surg 104:395–400
19. Moorehead RJ, Wong J (1990) Gangrene in esophageal substitutes after resection and bypass procedures for carcinoma of the esophagus. Hepatogastroenterology 37:364–367
20. Moreno-Gonzales E et al (1992) Esophageal resection through a translaparotomic-transcervical approach. Ann Ital Chir 63:33–37
21. Orringer MB et al (1988) Agressive treatment of chylothorax complicating transhiatal esophagectomy without thoracotomy. Surgery 104:720–726
22. Orringer MB et al (1993) Transhiatal esophagectomy for benign and malignant disease. J Thorac Cardiovasc Surg 105:265–276
23. Peracchia A and Bardini R (1986) Total esophagectomy without thoracotomy; results of a European questionnaire GEEMO. Int Surg 71:171–175
24. Peracchia A et al (1993) Cancer of the cervical esophagus: extent of resection, short- and long-term results of surgery. In: Nabeya K et al (eds) Diseases of the esophagus. Springer, Berlin Heidelberg New York, pp 630–635

25. Peracchia A et al (1992) The short term complications of the surgical treatment of thoracic esophageal carcinoma. Ann Ital Chir 63:39–43
26. Pierie JPEN et al (1993) Incidence and management of benign anastomotic stricture after cervical oesophagogastrostomy. Br J Surg 80:471–474
27. Ribet M et al (1992) Oesophagectomie pour cancer malpighien évolué de l'oesophage thoracique. Anastomose oesophago-gastrique au cou ou dans le thorax? Ann Chir 46:905–911
28. Siewert JR et al (1988) En-bloc resection of the esophagus in esophageal cancer. Langenbecks Arch Chir 373:367–376
29. Wang LS et al (1992) Gastric substitution for resectable carcinoma of the esophagus: an analysis of 368 cases. Ann Thorac Surg 53:289–294
30. Zieren HU et al (1993) Prospective randomized study of one or two-layer anastomosis following oesophageal resection and cervical oesophagogastrostomy. Br J Surg 80:608–611
31. Zieren HU et al (1995) Soll beim Magenhochzug nach subtotaler Oesophagektomie mit oesophago-gastraler Anastomose am Hals eine Pyloroplastik duchgeführt werden? Eine prospektiv randomisierte Studie. Chirurg 66:319–325

Photodynamic Therapy

C. Ell, L. Gossner

Second Medical Department, Klinikum Wiesbaden (HSK), Wiesbaden, Germany

Abstract

Photodynamic therapy (PDT) is a treatment modality that utilizes a photosensitizing drug activated by laser-generated light and is proving effective for oncologic and nononcologic applications in the gastrointestinal tract. This article provides an overview of the most frequently used photosensitizers and clincal PDT studies in the upper gastrointestinal tract. In the future, the best indications for PDT in the esophagus will not comprise the palliative treatment of obstructing tumors but precancerous lesions such as Barrett's esophagus with or without dysplasia and early cancer. PDT might establish itself as a minimally invasive treatment alternative compared with surgery for high-grade dysplasia or early mucosal cancer of the esophagus.

Introduction

Reports concerning intraluminal photodynamic therapy in the gastrointestinal tract first began to appear as early as the late 1980s [1, 2] and were greeted with both enthusiasm and controversy. In that respect, little has changed even today. It is not that photodynamic therapy (PDT) has been outdated, nor that its technical potential has been fully exhausted, nor that it has been superseded by more modern procedures. On the contrary, PDT is still going through a dynamic process of development, improvement, and standardization.

In addition to its as yet incomplete methodological development, at least three other factors are obstructing the widespread clinical application of PDT. The first of these is legal approval. So far, PDT has only been approved for use – sometimes with significant restrictions – in a few countries. On the basis of a large multicenter study, the health authorities in the United States have approved the use of PDT with first-generation photosensitizers (Photofrin) only for the palliative treatment of advanced esophageal carcinoma [3]. In Japan, however, the same substance can be legally used for the treatment of early carcinomas as well. In Europe, approval of the photosensitizer Photo-

Recent Results in Cancer Research, Vol. 155

frin for use in the gastrointestinal tract has been given in the Netherlands and France, but not in Germany or the United Kingdom. No approvals have been granted for the more modern photosensitizers, such as aminolevulinic acid (ALA) – nor are they likely to be approved in the foreseeable future, due to the high costs of the approval procedure and the unsuitability of the substance for patenting. This means that clinicians using these substances are in a quite unsafe area, and that these photosensitizers should be used only under the strictest possible conditions.

The second important factor hindering the widespread use of PDT is the fact that the laser systems required for PDT are currently expensive to purchase and maintain. In Germany, at least, suitable laser systems capable of being used in everyday clinical practice by physicians and nurses cost between $150,000 and $225,000. In addition, there is the cost of the fiber systems, applicators, and the necessary dye exchanges. Since the available lasers are not tunable, they could easily become unsuitable if a different photosensitizer were to be used, since each photosensitizer has a specific absorption maximum.

The third factor standing in the way of PDT is the lack of demonstrated areas of application in large numbers of patients. One ideal form of treatment in this respect would be *Helicobacter pylori* eradication using photodynamic irradiation, which has been successfully achieved experimentally [4]. But it would be completely divorced from clinical reality to believe that this type of intraluminal treatment, even if it was clinically effective, would ever be accepted or would be economical.

Palliative treatment of stenotic tumors of the esophagus, stomach, and colon does not provide any hopeful prospects for widespread use of photodynamic procedures, either. Although the multicenter American study mentioned above showed that fewer treatment sessions were required with PDT in comparison with Nd:YAG laser therapy, and that there was also a lower perforation rate, the economic arguments are not convincing here in view of the high cost of PDT and the short life expectancy in this group of patients [3]. The American health authorities have just approved PDT exclusively for palliation, but in clinical reality there are in fact simpler thermodestruction procedures and, particularly in the esophagus, mature techniques using self-expanding metal endoprostheses are available for simpler and more effective palliation [5].

With regard to the palliative treatment of malignant stenoses of the bile ducts using PDT, one complete paper and one abstract have been published, reporting small numbers of cases. However, these require confirmation in larger studies – preferably multicenter prospective and comparative ones – before this treatment procedure can be seriously recommended. There appear to be potential problems with the light application and dosimetry, which are carried out without direct endoscopic control. The high porphyrin concentration in the liver still needs to be borne in mind [6, 7]. Nor is PDT likely to be of any significance in the treatment of villous rectal adenomas and flat papillary adenomas, due to the alternative treatment procedures that are available and the low numbers of cases [8].

In Western countries, early gastric carcinoma is being diagnosed endoscopically with increasing frequency, and patients are receiving local curative treatment (and not only in inoperable cases). When prior staging examinations are carried out, the histological and endoscopic ultrasound findings can be used to identify with a high degree of certainty those patients able to benefit from local curative treatment. Particularly when endoscopic mucosal resection is not possible or is not successful, PDT represents a good alternative [9, 10]. In our group at least, the photosensitizer meta-tetrahydroxyphenylchlorine (mTHPC) has proved its value. With no significant morbidity and, in particular, with no cases of perforation, complete tumor destruction was achieved in approximately 80% of patients treated. The follow-up period is clearly limited, and the results achieved are therefore preliminary. Particularly in tumors that cannot be clearly located endoscopically ("biopsy carcinoma"), photodynamic treatment of larger areas using mTHPC - or even with ALA, which is much less problematic in clinical practice - is a procedure that is fundamentally different from thermoablation methods and mucosectomy, and should therefore be considered as a potential treatment option.

The most frequent indication for PDT in the future may be Barrett's esophagus. However, PDT of any type is also in competition with the various methods of thermoablation and endoscopic mucosal resection (EMR) as well (Table 1). The incidence of the diagnosis of Barrett's esophagus has rapidly increased in recent years [11]. There is nowadays also a broad awareness of the metaplasia–dysplasia–carcinoma sequence, and this in part explains the increasing rate of diagnosis. In a more detailed discussion, it is useful to distinguish between Barrett's metaplasia with or without dysplasia, on the one hand, and severe dysplasia or early Barrett's carcinoma on the other. The precondition for local endoscopic therapy for Barrett's esophagus with or without mild dysplasia should be that the method used allows complete ablation of the undesirable epithelium

Table 1. Endoscopic techniques for local treatment of Barrett's syndrome

1	Thermocoagulation
	Laser
	Nd:YAG laser
	Argon laser
	Electrocoagulation
	Monopolar (e.g., electrohydrothermoprobe, EHT)
	Multipolar
	Argon beamer
2	Photodynamic therapy (PDT) with:
	Hematoporphyrin
	5-Aminolevulinic acid
	Chlorine (e.g., mTHPC)
3	Endoscopic mucosal resection (EMR)
	Snare resection without saline injection
	Snare resection with saline injection
	Snare resection with "suck and cut" technique

Table 2. Results of local endoscopic therapy of Barrett's syndrome (published as full papers in Western journals)

Reference	Method	Barrett's without HGD/early cancer	Barrett's with HGD/early cancer	Patients (*n*)	Complete remission (*n*)
Berenson (1993) [12]	Argon laser	+	–	10	9
Sampliner (1996) [14]	Electro-coagulation	+	–	10	9
Barham (1997) [15]	KTP laser	+	–	11	6
Gossner (1998) [16]	KTP laser	– (4)	+ (6)	10	10
Laukka (1995) [17]	PDT	+	–	5	5
Overholt (1995) [18]	PDT	–	+	24	20
Gossner (1995) [19]	PDT-ALA	–	+	5	4
Barr (1996) [21]	PDT-ALA	–	+	5	5
Gossner (1998) [22]	PDT-ALA	–	+	32	27
Takeshita (1997) [23]	EMR	–	+	56	56

ALA, 5-aminolevulinic acid; EMR, endoscopic mucosal resection; HGD, high-grade dysplasia; KTP, potassium titanyl phosphate; PDT, photodynamic therapy.

and complete restitution of orthotopic epithelium. The existing data do not yet allow firm conclusions to be drawn (Table 2). However, the data on the use of PDT in the treatment of Barrett's epithelium seem to be slightly better than those for thermoablation [12–26]. In addition, ablation using the spot effects of thermal procedures – whether laser coagulation or thermocoagulation – produces varying depths and not infrequently causes tissue destruction that also affects the submucosa. By contrast, PDT with ALA is limited in its destructive effects on the mucosa, as has been adequately shown in animal experiments [26]. In this respect, ALA–PDT has a clear advantage over thermocoagulation procedures. In addition, suitable light applicators can be used to achieve homogeneous and circumferential irradiation in a single session, over a length of up to 8 cm [27–29]. Summing up, it appears that ALA–PDT treatment of Barrett's mucosa with or without mild dysplasia has basic advantages over the alternative procedures, although there is still a lack of adequate clinical confirmation. In addition, it has not been adequately confirmed whether ablation techniques in general do in fact provide an economically defensible form of carcinoma prevention.

Although the case numbers concerned are smaller, the question of how to deal with Barrett's epithelium and severe dysplasia or early carcinoma is of much greater clinical relevance. The gold standard is undoubtedly still radical surgery, with partial gastric and esophageal resection. However, careful study of the published surgical data shows that there are good arguments for local therapy. On the one hand, there are the considerable morbidity and mortality rates associated with radical surgery, which even in high-grade dysplasia or early carcinoma in Barrett's esophagus amount to between 30% and 50%, or 3% and 5%, respectively. The available surgical and pathoanatomical data indicate that the risk of lymph-node metastasis in high-grade dysplasia and in mucosal early carcinoma is almost zero. In any case, it is lower than the mortality rates with surgery. In choosing a local treatment procedure, endoscopic mucosal resection is undoubtedly the first option. However, EMR can only be used if the malignant lesions can be clearly located. In addition, the resection cannot exceed a certain size, and in multifocal conditions, too, EMR is not yet a suitable form of primary therapy. This suggests one potential indication for PDT: whenever a biopsy has demonstrated malignancy or severe dysplasia but macroscopic identification is unclear, and in cases of long Barrett's segments with advanced histological changes, PDT should be considered as a primary form of local treatment.

With the usual form of PDT, strictures occurred in up to half of the patients, but all of these were easy to treat endoscopically [15, 30]. In Overholt's group, this relatively aggressive form of treatment was followed by complete remission in all patients, and this was also confirmed during a follow-up period of up to 5 years [15]. Using the "milder" form of ALA-PDT, which is limited to selective destruction of the mucosa, Barr's group and our own group achieved long-term complete remission in all cases of high-grade dysplasia. Long-term remission was seen in only around 75% of patients who already had early carcinoma, however [16, 17]. When the mucosa has thickened by more than 2 mm, i.e., when mucosal changes are already visible macroscopically, ALA-PDT is very likely to be inadequate, and a more intensive form of PDT should be used instead - for example, with mTHPC as the photosensitizer. The data on PDT in severe dysplasia and early carcinoma in Barrett's esophagus are very promising, but due to the small numbers of patients overall and the very short follow-up period, a conclusive assessment of the value of the method is not yet possible.

With regard to the use of PDT in the treatment of early squamous-cell carcinoma in the esophagus, there have also only been very few reports so far, at least from the Western hemisphere [30]. When ALA is used as the photosensitizer, all of the patients with high-grade dysplasia who were treated in our group experienced complete remission, but only about half of those with confirmed early carcinoma had remissions. No significant side effects of the treatment were observed [30]. By contrast, the results of PDT with mTHPC of the Lausanne group were better with regard to complete remission, although this was at the expense of increased morbidity. Summing up, PDT may therefore be of significance in the future for the treatment of high-risk patients with early squamous-cell carcinoma, since, in comparison with radical surgery or aggressive chemoradiotherapy, PDT represents a form of minimally invasive treatment. Here, too, however, the search for optimal irradiation conditions is not yet complete.

In conclusion, PDT is a fascinating concept, which will continue to occupy many research groups around the world in the coming years. Although a widespread clinical application for the method has not yet emerged, there are good prospects that PDT will be able to establish itself at major gastroenterological centers as an endoscopic procedure with few or no side effects in the treatment of Barrett's esophagus (severe dysplasia and early carcinoma) and, in selected cases, also for the treatment of early squamous-cell carcinoma and early gastric carcinoma.

References

1. McCaugham JS, Nims TA, Guy JT, Laufmann LR (1989) Photodynamic therapy for oesophageal tumours. Arch Surg 124:74–80
2. Thomas RJ, Abbott K, Bhatal PS, Morstyn H (1987) High-dose photoradiation of oesophageal cancers. Ann Surg 206:193–199
3. Lightdale CJ, Heier SK, Marcon NE et al (1995) Photodynamic therapy with porfimer sodium versus thermal ablation therapy with Nd:YAG laser for palliation of esophageal cancer: a multicenter randomized trial. Gastrointest Endosc 42:507–512
4. Milson CE, Wilson M, Bown SG (1996) Ex vivo treatment of gastric Helicobacter infection by photodynamic therapy. J Photochem Photobiol 32:S946
5. Ell C, May A (1997) Self-expanding metal stents for the palliation of stenosing tumors of the esophagus and cardia. Endoscopy 29:392–398
6. Ortner A, Ernst H, Lochs H (1998) Photodynamic therapy of malignant common bile duct stenoses. Gastroenterology 114:9–14
7. Berr E, Mössner P (1997) Photodynamische Therapie von cholangiocellulären Carcinomen (abstract). Z Gastroenterol 35:691
8. Bown SG (1994) Photodynamic therapy of villous adenoma of the rectosigmoid. Endoscopy 26:234–242
9. Kato H, Kawaguchi M, Konaka C (1986) Evaluation of photodynamic therapy in gastric cancer. Laser Med Sci 1:67–74
10. Ell C, Gossner L, May A et al (1998) Photodynamic therapy of early gastric cancer with mTHPC. Gut 43:345–349
11. Prach AT, MacDonald TA, Hopwood DA, Johnston DA (1997) Increasing incidence of Barrett's oesophagus: education, enthusiasm, or epidemiology? Lancet 350:933
12. Berenson MM, Johnson TD, Markowitz NR et al (1993) Restoration of squamous mucosa after ablation of Barrett's esophageal epithelium. Gastroenterology 104:1686–1691
13. Sampliner RE, Hixon LJ, Fennerty MB, Garewal HS (1993) Regression of Barrett's esophagus by laser ablation in an anacid environment. Dig Dis Sci 38:365–368
14. Sampliner RE, Fennerty MB, Garewal HS (1996) Reversal of Barrett's esophagus with acid suppression and multipolar electrocoagulation: preliminary results. Gastrointest Endosc 44:523–525
15. Barham OP, Jonas RL, Biddlestone LR et al (1997) Photothermal laser ablation of Barrett's oesophagus: endoscopic and histological evidence of squamous re-epithelialization. Gut 41:281–284
16. Gossner L, May A, Stolte M, Seitz G, Ell C (1999) KTP-laser destruction of dysplasia and early cancer in columnar-lined Barrett's esophagus. Gastrointest Endosc 49:8–12
17. Laukka MA, Wang KK (1995) Initial results using low-dose photodynamic therapy in the treatment of Barrett's esophagus. Gastrointest Endosc 42:59–63
18. Overholt OF, Panjehpour M (1995) Barrett's esophagus: photodynamic therapy for ablation of dysplasia, reduction of specialized mucosa, and treatment of superficial esophageal cancer. Gastrointest Endosc 42:64–69

19. Gossner L, Sroka R, Hahn EG, Ell C (1995) Photodynamic therapy: successful destruction of gastrointestinal cancer after oral administration of aminolaevulinic acid. Gastrointest Endosc 41:55
20. Overholt BF, Panjehpour M (1996) Photodynamic therapy for Barrett's esophagus: clinical update. Am J Gastroenterol 91:1719–1722
21. Barr H, Shepherd NA, Dix A et al (1996) Eradication of high-grade dysplasia in columnar-lined (Barrett's) oesophagus by photodynamic therapy with endogenously generated protoporphyrin IX. Lancet 348:584–585
22. Gossner L, Stolte M, Sroka R, Ell C (1998) Photodynamic ablation of high-grade dysplasia and early cancer in Barrett's esophagus by means of 5-aminolevulinic acid. Gastroenterology 114:448–455
23. Takeshita K, Inoue H, Saeki I et al (1997) Endoscopic treatment of early oesophageal or gastric cancer. Gut 40:123–127
24. Soehendra N, Binmoeller KF, Bohnacker S et al (1987) Endoscopic snare mucosectomy in the esophagus without any additional equipment: a simple technique for resection of flat early cancer. Endoscopy 29:380–383
25. Sibille A, Lambert R, Souquet JC et al (1995) Long-term survival after photodynamic therapy for esophageal cancer. Gastroenterology 108:337–344
26. Loh CS, MacRobert AJ, Krasner N, Bown SG (1996) Mucosal ablation using photodynamic therapy for the treatment of dysplasia: an experimental study in the normal rat stomach. Gut 38:71–78
27. Monnier F, Savary JM, van den Bergh H (1996) Photodetection and photodynamic therapy of early squamous cell carcinoma of the pharynx, esophagus and tracheo-bronchial tree. Laser Med Sci 5:149–159
28. Overholt BF, Panjehpour M, DeNovo RC (1996) Balloon photodynamic therapy for esophageal cancer. Lasers Surg Med 18:248–252
29. Gossner L, Sroka R, Ell C (1999) A new long-range through-the-scope balloon applicator for photodynamic therapy in the esophagus and cardia. Endoscopy (in press)
30. Gossner L, Stolte M, Sroka R, Ell C (1998) Photodynamische Therapie von Plattenepithelfrühkarzinomen und schweren plattenepithelialen Dysplasien der Speiseröhre mit 5-Aminolävulinsäure. Z Gastroenterol 36:19–26

Endoscopic Mucosectomy: An Alternative Treatment for Superficial Esophageal Cancer

R. Lambert

Department of Digestive Diseases, Hospital Edouard Herriot,
F-69374 Lyon Cedex 03, France

Abstract

Recent trends in the management of superficial esophageal cancer consist of improved detection, pretherapeutic staging and reliable criteria for curative endoscopic therapy. The endoscopic treatment is legitimate when the cancer is at an early stage, intra-epithelial or microinvasive (m1 or m2) and N0. Submucosal cancer should not be treated with a curative intent by endotherapy. Concerning squamous cell cancer, the oriental and occidental pathologists include high-grade dysplasia in the same group as intramucosal cancer. The distinction is however maintained for adenocarcinoma in the Barrett's esophagus. Indications of endoscopic rather than surgical treatment rely on: (1) the small size of the tumor (not more than 2 cm in diameter); (2) the endoscopic morphology in the type 0 of the Japanese classification with the flat subtypes IIa and IIb rather than type IIc – there is high risk of submucosal invasion for the polypoid (type I) or ulcerated superficial cancer (type III); and (3) the endoscopic ultrasound staging, with confirmed integrity of the hyperechoic submucosal layer. The high-frequency (20 MHz) miniprobe is preferred to the standard (7.5 MHz) instrument. The elective procedure for tumor eradication is endoscopic mucosectomy. The technique is associated with a 6.8% risk of severe complications (hemorrhage or perforation) and a recurrence rate of 3%–7%. The 5-year survival rate is similar to that of surgery (over 80%). In the small group of patients with superficial esophageal cancer (less than 10% of the disease) endoscopic treatment may now be proposed in about 30% of cases, surgery is preferred for submucosal cancer and for neoplasia with a large surface. Areas of high-grade dysplasia in the Barrett's esophagus offer a new and increasing sector of indications. The concurrent endoscopic procedure of destruction – photodynamic therapy – is preferred for the destruction of lesions with poorly delineated limits.

Recent Results in Cancer Research, Vol. 155

Introduction

With respect to the worldwide deaths from cancer in 1996 (WHO, Geneva, 1997), esophageal cancer ranks fifth. The poor prognosis of the tumor is shown when comparing the annual incidence, prevalence (5 years) and mortality: the figures are very similar. Indeed, in 1996, the estimated number of new cases in the world was 480 000, slightly higher than the estimated number of deaths (456 000). In tumor registries, the overall 5 year relative survival rate varies from 5% to 8% in most countries; the crude survival rate would be lower. In epidemiology statistics, around 85% of esophageal cancer occurs in developing countries with the highest risk in the Asian belt, and a dramatic increase in esophageal adenocarcinoma occurs in occidental countries [1–4] in relation to columnar metaplasia in the Barrett's esophagus. Squamous neoplasia represents over 95% of cases of esophageal cancer in Asiatic countries and in non-Caucasian races; while, in western countries and in Caucasians, adenocarcinoma is observed in 40%–50% of cases.

Most cases of esophageal cancer are detected at an advanced stage with a very poor prognosis and recent trends are associated with the contribution of the chemoradiation protocol. Only a small percentage of cases are detected at an early stage of evolution when the tumor is superficial. The recent trends concern the contribution of endoscopic ultrasonography to staging and the reliability of an endoscopic curative treatment, with a strict indication and protocol.

The Rationale for Endoscopic Treatment of Superficial Cancer

Endoscopic treatment is equivalent to a localized tissue destruction or resection; the radical cure will be obtained only at the early stage of neoplasia, in the absence of regional and systemic lymphatic or vascular invasion. This situation corresponds to intramucosal dysplasia or cancer; invasion of the submucosa or the muscularis propria corresponds to advanced cancer; the tumor at this stage shall not be cured by a local intraparietal intervention. Therefore, the rationale of endoscopic curative treatment is based on a safe pretherapeutic estimation of the pathology; this depends on endoscopy and endoscopic ultrasonography.

Anatomical Classification of Esophageal Cancer

The classification established in 1992 by the Japanese Society for Esophageal Diseases [5] concerns the squamous cell cancer type in the esophagus. Superficial esophageal cancer is a T1 tumor in the TNM classification; the depth of invasion is limited to the mucosa or the submucosa [6–11]. The definition of early stage is intramucosal cancer without lymphatic metastases. This corresponds to intraepithelial tumors (m1, N0) and to microinvasive tumors with effraction of the basal membrane (m2, N0) and to some, but not all, tumors reaching the muscularis mucosae (m3, N0). Overall, the percentage of N+ tumors is very small (around 3%–5%) in esophageal intramucosal cancer. When there is penetration in the submucosa (sm), the tumor is considered as advanced cancer with a rate of positive lymph nodes around 35%–40% [6]; this concerns the various grades of the submucosal invasion (sm1, sm2, sm3). A safe indication of curative endoscopic treatment is limited to intramucosal cancer, and most probably to the subtypes m1 and m2 [8, 9]. Concerning squamous neoplasia, Oriental and occidental pathologists agree to consider high-grade dysplasia and intraepithelial cancer in the same group.

The Japanese classification may be adapted for the adenocarcinoma tumor type, but with some simplification. Indeed, the distinction between intraepithelial and microinvasive is not relevant for a columnar mucosa. Therefore, intramucosal glandular cancer is localized with a very low risk of lymphatic extension and may be treated at endoscopy. Submucosal glandular cancer should not be treated this way, owing to the risk of lymphatic extension. Concerning columnar neoplasia, the distinction between high-grade dysplasia and cancer persists. Oriental and occidental pathologists differ however in their interpretation of cancer. Oriental pathologists rely on cytological and architectural criteria, occidental pathologists rely on criteria of invasion. This is why around 30% of cases classified as intramucosal cancer in Japan will be classified as high-grade dysplasia in the western world. However, both groups agree to cancer classification when there is invasion of the submucosa.

Endoscopic Evaluation of Superficial Cancer

The detection of early neoplasia requires a careful analysis of the mucosal lining of the esophagus, looking for slight changes in color and relief [11]; forceps biopsies in the abnormal area will confirm the diagnosis. Elevated areas are whitish; depressed areas are more colored in red. Chromoscopy is helpful using a spray catheter with a 2.5% solution of lugol – squamous neoplastic areas remain unstained and contrast with the dark brown appearance of the normal mucosa. The indigocarmine solution diluted at 0.5% enhances the contrast architecture and is helpful in the analysis of dysplasia in the columnar metaplasia in the distal esophagus.

Neoplastic lesions with a superficial pattern are called stage 0 in the Japanese endoscopic classification [5]. The prediction of the superficial depth of invasion depends essentially of the surface pattern. In the polypoid type I and the ulcerated type III, invasion of the submucosa is frequent; therefore, a local endoscopic treatment is probably unsafe. The flat pattern type II is described with three subtypes: IIa or elevated, IIb or flat and IIc or depressed. The types IIa and IIb have less potential for submucosal infiltration than the type IIc. Finally, the mixed pattern IIa+IIc is suggestive of a deep infiltration in the submucosa. The extension of the neoplastic area is just as important in the analysis. The risk of invasion in the submucosa usually increases with the surface extension, with the exception of some superficial spreading types. Furthermore large surfaces are not compatible with a safe complete destruction and the chances of complications are higher.

In function of both parameters (surface extension and surface morphology), the safe indications of curative endotherapy in the esophagus are diameter up to 2 cm (or 30% of esophageal circumference) for neoplastic areas with the subtype IIa or IIb and diameter up to 1 cm for lesions with the subtype IIc [9].

Endoscopic Ultrasonographic Evaluation of Superficial Cancer

The endoscopic ultrasonic (EUS) exploration aims to assess the depth of invasion of the esophageal wall by the tumor and, in complement, the presence of malignant regional lymph nodes [11–13]. EUS exploration is conducted with a first objective: the distinction between superficial T1 cancer (limited to the mucosa and the submucosa) and the more advanced cancer T2, T3 and T4. The second objective is adapted to the exploration of the columnar lining: the distinction between intramucosal cancer and cancer with an extension in the submucosa. Finally in the squamous cell lining, a further distinction would require the separation of m1 and m2 cancer, m3 cancer and sm1 cancer; this requires identification of the muscularis mucosae as a hypoechoic layer. The elective indications of curative endotherapy are limited to the first group (m1, m2).

With conventional EUS at 12 MHz, the distinction of T1 versus non-T1 tumor is reliable with 90% confidence [12–14]. The distinction is based on the integrity of the third hyperechoic layer, corresponding to the submucosa. However, the separation between a tumor strictly confined in the mucosa and a tumor penetrating in the submucosa without outpassing this layer is not as reliable, and the identification of the muscularis mucosae is rather uncertain. This introduces a weak point in the rational for elective indications of curative endotherapy. However, there is considerable progress in the technology of EUS with high-frequency (12–20 MHz) US miniprobes [15–17]. The miniprobe passing through the operative channel of the scope is placed under view control in contact with the lesion. The acoustic liaison is ensured by a transparent plastic bag (condom model) filled with water. A nine-layer diagram is obtained with identification of the muscularis mucosae as a fourth hypoechoic layer. In a recent series, an 84% accuracy in the detection of intraepithelial cancer was reported [16]. There is no doubt that intramucosal cancer shall be identified with confidence in the near future.

Adequate Indications of Curative Endotherapy in Esophageal Cancer

The elective indications, proposed as an alternative to surgery, inclusive in patients with no operative contraindications, are summarized as follows:
- Surface morphology of the lesions with the subtype IIa, IIb, IIc
- Diameters up to 2 cm (or 1 cm for the depressed lesion)
- No suspect regional lymph node at EUS exploration
- Complete integrity of the third (hyperechoic) layer at 12 MHz with the conventional echoendoscope.

However, the staging with the high-frequency miniprobe is more and more often required. For patients at risk of requiring surgery and with a poor health status relative to age or an associated disease, the indications may be enlarged with respect to surface morphology and depth of invasion.

Endoscopic Procedures for Tumor Eradication

The procedures adapted to curative endotherapy are the resection or the destruction of the neoplastic area. The endoscopic mucosal resection or EMR [18–25] has a major advantage: a specimen is available for staging and treatment decision may be altered, according to the results of pathology. Actually, the EMR is a complete biopsy technique and may as well be a complete treatment when the elective criteria are met.

The procedures of destruction rely either on a thermal reaction or on a photobiological reaction. Various devices have been used (plasma argon coagulator [26], gold probe, heater probe); however, the Nd:YAG laser is the most powerful and the most employed device. Non-thermal procedures rely on the concentration of a photosensitizer in the tumor [27–30]. The agent is activated by a photon laser beam after an interval of time: Photofrin (a hematoporphyrin derivative, dose 2 mg/kg body weight) is still the reference product [30] with either squamous cell cancer or dysplasia in the Barrett's esophagus. Other agents have been employed, such as chlorin and 5 aminolevulinic acid [29]. The later agent has been proposed in the treatment of dysplasia in the Barrett's esophagus.

The EMR is without doubt the elective procedure in curative endotherapy of esophageal cancer, but there is still room for procedures of destruction, because they are easier to perform. The thermal destruction of small neoplastic lesions with the Nd:YAG laser is convenient for the destruction of sessile and thick neoplastic areas in patients at risk of surgery; furthermore, as shown by various teams in Japan, it may be used to complete the EMR when the access to the lesion is difficult. The non-thermal photobiological procedures have indications in the treatment of flat, occult, poorly delineated neoplastic areas, such as observed in columnar neoplasia. A new sector of elective indications is opening with the treatment of high-grade dysplasia in the Barrett's esophagus.

The Technique for EMR

The technique of EMR is accessible to any team familiar with interventional endoscopy; the procedure is similar in the esophagus, stomach, duodenum or colon. A progressive simplification occurred: EMR was initially performed with the help of two operative channels, one for the snare, the other for a grasping forceps. This was achieved either using a double channel scope or a single channel scope passing through an overtube with another channel [22]. The simplest procedure, allowing more diffusion has been proposed by H. Inoue, which requires a single channel cap-fitted endoscope; the procedure derives from the ligator kit [20, 21] employing aspiration in combination with the lifting of the lesion after submucosal injection of saline. The lifting helps to snare the mucosa and has a prognostic value. The invasion of the submucosa is probable when the lesion is not lifted. An alternative procedure of mucosal resection uses either a simple snare [23] or the standard material of the endoscopic ligator kit instead of the transparent cap. The elastic ring is placed just distal to the line of resection [24, 25]. This should be used only when the specific transparent cap is not available. The following steps must be carefully followed during the intervention:

- Just before resection, the morphology of the lesion should be analyzed with care and the limits of the neoplastic area are marked with white cauterization dots with a 3-mm safety margin – the lesion is then lifted above the surface with saline submucosal injection at the periphery in three to four distinct points.
- The resection itself is performed using a thin pediatric crescent snare placed along the distal ring of the transparent cap, adhering to the tip of the scope – the aspirated neoplastic surface enters into the snare and is sectioned at distance of the cap. The resected segment is then collected. Piecemeal resection with successive lifted, aspirated and collected segments is possible, until the resection is complete.
- After the resection, a final control of the resected surface is made, hemostatic clips are placed eventually and the specimen is prepared for pathology with reconstitution of the total surface of the lesion pinned in a cardboard.

EMR and Multimodal Protocols

When the treatment option is a curative endoscopic procedure (resection or tumor destruction), it should be performed in monotherapy. The safety of the procedure depends on the adequate selection of the indication and an appropriate methodology. The success, or failure, is assessed by the biopsies at the endoscopic control after a few weeks. The regional (radiation) and systemic (chemotherapy) therapeutic agents are not helpful for a localized lesion. Furthermore, their application, is a source of systemic and local side effects. The inflammatory response at the tumor site is often a source of confusion in the evaluation of the tumor response as complete or incomplete.

The Results of EMR

Most data concerning curative endotherapy of superficial cancer in the upper digestive tract are found in the Japanese literature, and most data are on stomach cancer. The results concern the tolerance and side effects or complications of the procedure and the rate of complete tumor response in the short term and finally the 5 year survival. This is a relatively new method and the results are not yet evidence based as soundly as in surgery. The Japanese school considers that the 5 year survival rate after EMR varies between 95% and 100% with a recurrence rate of 3%–7%. The endoscopic resection is proposed in around 25% of all early upper gastrointestinal cancers. Concerning stomach cancer, strictly parallel survival curves after EMR or surgery have been produced since 1993 [19]. Another series [20] in 1994 confirmed the safety of the procedure; the rate of complete resection in elective indications reached 89% for the elevated type (up to 2 cm) and 83% for the depressed type (up to 1 cm).

Concerning esophageal intramucosal cancer, a similar 5 year survival rate was observed in 1995 [18] for EMR, the endoscopic treatment (86%) and for conventional surgery (83.2%). Noteworthy, the patients were treated by the same operators. In this series, the rate of EMR complications was 12.9% during the early period and 7.2% later. Severe complications included bleeding, perforation and later stenosis. More recently [9], the results of the treatment of superficial cancer were reviewed in a meta-analysis (143 institutions with a total 2418 patients); the questionnaire concerns the period 1990–1994; the indication of EMR was limited to m1 and m2 cancer in 76% of institutions. Complications occurred in 6.8% of cases. It is concluded that local resection of esophageal cancer is a treatment of choice for tumors limited to m1 or m2. In another series [10], 56 treated cases were all alive and a good epithelialization occurred without complication after EMR.

The Endoscopic Treatment of Dysplasia in Barrett's Esophagus

The oriental studies on curative endotherapy of tumors in the esophagus concern exclusively the squamous cell cancer type. In the Western World, neoplasia (intramucosal cancer or high-grade dysplasia) arising in the columnar metaplastic mucosa is another tumor type. The curative endotherapy of high-grade columnar dysplasia deserves to be encouraged relative to the dramatic increase in the incidence of adenocarcinoma in the esophagus and at the cardia; more and more individuals with a Barrett's esophagus are becoming involved in surveillance programs. The finding of high-grade dysplasia suggests a high risk for either an association with or a progression to a lesion with a confirmed adenocarcinoma. Nowadays, the therapeutic alternative for high-grade dysplasia is between esophagectomy (a aggressive procedure) and surveillance (often ineffective); this is why curative endotherapy should be preferred if it proves active. Actually, the treatment of dysplasia in the Barrett's esophagus is based either on thermal procedures of destruction or on non-thermal procedures with photodynamic therapy. Due to the occult morphology of the lesions and their unconspicuous limits, photodynamic therapy is the more adapted endoscopic procedure. However, there is room for EMR, either in complement with PDT or as the elective treatment of small neoplastic areas. When dysplasia is classified with a moderate grade, errors with inflammation are common, and biopsies are repeated 3 months later after a therapeutic trial with proton-pump inhibitors. If moderate dysplasia is confirmed, recent trends consider treatment rather than surveillance. Promising early results have been recently published, using either photofrin or 5-aminolevulinic acid [29, 30]. Finally, there has been some attempts at endoscopic treatment of metaplasia in the Barrett's esophagus. This is based on the following assumption: there is no significant regression of metaplasia with acid inhibition alone (achieved by surgery or proton pump inhibitors). On the contrary, if the metaplastic mucosa is destroyed, healing in an acid environment occurs with reversion to squamous epithelium [31, 32]. It has, therefore, been proposed to eradicate the metaplasia in association with prolonged acid inhibition using either thermal (gold probe, argon coagulator) or non-thermal (PDT) procedures. However, this should be considered with caution because the complete destruction of the metaplastic area is more than uncertain when the segment is long with a great surface area; furthermore, during the follow-up, re-growth of glands with intestinal metaplasia occurs under a reverted normal squamous epithelium [29]. The high cost of prolonged acid inhibition at high dose in maintenance therapy is another objection.

Conclusions

In synthesis, there is room for endoscopic procedures in curative treatment of esophagogastric cancer, but the concept is still confined to Japan – other countries share skepticism either regarding the existence of or the benefit in treating such early lesions. The safety and efficacy of EMR in stomach cancer is based on large numbers and a long observation period. Concerning esophageal cancer, the Japanese experience is based on squamous cell cancer with much smaller numbers and a shorter period of observation. In the Western world, lesions fulfilling the Japanese criteria are considered as rare in the stomach and also in the esophagus. A significant increase requires a change in the policy of screening with endoscopy. A promising field for curative endotherapy is the columnar neoplasia, including altogether the premalignant high-grade dysplasia and the intramucosal cancer in the lower esophagus and at the cardia.

The accepted principles of the Japanese school of gastroenterology must be adopted: endoscopic screening for early cancer is encouraged in asymptomatic persons. A special attention is given during endoscopy to minor changes in the mucosal surface (architecture, color) and the practice of chromoscopy is systematic. The flat neoplastic areas (the so-called 0 type) are carefully examined and classified in sub-types of prognostic value with prediction of the depth of invasion. The diameter of the lesion enters into the criteria of inclusion or rejection. The invasion in depth is controlled at EUS. Finally, in Japan, the simultaneous practice by upper-gastrointestinal specialists of interventional endoscopy and surgery avoids competition between specialists, and the comparison of results is easier. The preparation and stretching of the specimen for pathology is carried by the endoscopist. In the Western world, the elective endoscopic treatment must gain acceptance as an alternative to conventional surgery, as suggested in recent literature [34, 35].

References

1. Daly JM, Karnell LH, Menck HR (1996) National cancer data base report on esophageal carcinoma. Cancer 78:1820–1828
2. Spechler SJ, Goyal RK (1996) The columnar lined esophagus, intestinal metaplasia and Norman Barrett. Gastroenterology 111:614–621
3. Spechler SJ (1997) Esophageal columnar metaplasia (Barrett's) Gastrointest Endosc Clin N Am 7:1–18
4. Nandurkar S, Talley NJ, Martin CJ, Ng THK, Adams S (1997) Short segment Barrett's oesophagus: prevalence, diagnosis and associations. Gut 40:710–715
5. Japanese Society for Esophageal Diseases (1992) Guidelines for the clinical and pathologic studies on carcinoma of the esophagus, 8th edn. Kanehara, Tokyo
6. Nabeya K, Hanaoka T, Li S, Nyumura T (1993) What is the ideal treatment for early esophageal cancer. Endoscopy 25:670–671
7. Kitamura K, Kuwano H, Yasuda M, Sonoda K, Sumiyoshi K, Tsutsui S, Kitamura M, Sugimachi K (1966) What is the earliest malignant lesion, in the esophagus? Cancer 77:1614–1619
8. Kodama M, Kakegawa T (1996) Treatment of superficial carcinoma of the esophagus. A review of responses to questionnaire on superficial carcinoma of the esophagus, collected at the 49th conference of JSED. Nippon Gekka Gakkai Zasshi 97(8):683–690
9. Kodama M, Kakegawa T (1998) Treatment of superficial carcinoma of the esophagus. A review of responses to questionnaire on superficial carcinoma of the esophagus, in Japan. Surgery 123:432–439
10. Takeshita K, Tani M, Inoue H, Saeki I, Hayashi S, Honda T, Kando F, Saito N, Endo M (1997) Endoscopic treatment of early esophageal or gastric cancer. Gut 40:123–127
11. Endo M, Kawano T (1997) Detection and classification of early squamous cell esophageal cancer. Dis Esophag 10:155–158
12. Caletti G, Ferrari A (1996) Endoscopic ultrasonography. Endoscopy 28 156–173
13. Pollack BJ, Chak A, Sivak MV Jr (1996) Endoscopic ultrasonography. Semin Oncol 23:336–346
14. Fockens P, Van Lanschot JJB, Tytgat GNT (1996) The role of endosonography in esophageal carcinoma: who should get it, who should do it? Scand J Gastroenterol 31[Suppl 218]:82–85
15. Menzel J, Domschke W, Brambs HJ et al (1996) Miniprobe ultrasound of the upper gastrointestional tract. 1995 state of the art and perspectives. Ultraschall Med 17:143–148
16. Murata Y, Suzuki S, Ota M, Mitsunaga A, Hayashi K, Yoshida K, Ide H (1996) Small ultrasonic probes for determination of the depth of superficial esophageal cancer. Gastrointest Endosc 44:23–28
17. Yanai H, Yoshida T, Harada T, Matsumoto Y, Nishiaki M, Shidemiotsu T, Tada M, Okita K, Kawano T, Nagasaki S (1996) Endoscopic ultrasonography of superficial esophageal

cancers using a thin ultrasound probe system equipped with switchable radial and linear scanning modes. Gastrointest Endosc 44:578–582

18. Yoshida M, Hanashi T, momma K Yamada Y, Sakaki N, Koike M, Takisawa T, Kawamura T (1995) Endoscopic mucosal resection for radical treatment of esophageal cancer (in Japanese). Gan To Kagaku Ryoho 22:847–854
19. Tada M, Murakami A, Karita M,Yanai H, Okita K (1993) Endoscopic resection of early gastric cancer. Endoscopy 25:445–450
20. Takekoshi T, Baba Y, 0ta H, Kato Y, Yanagisawa A, Tagaki K, Noguchi Y (1994) Endoscopic resection of early gastric carcinoma: results of a retrospective analysis of 308 cases. Endoscopy 26:352–358
21. Tada M, Inoue H, Yabata E, Okabe S, Endo M (1996) Colonic resection using a transparent cap fitted endoscope. Gastrointest Endosc 44:63–65
22. Inoue M, Shiozaki H, Tamura S, Monden M (1996) Endoscopic mucosal resection for early esophageal cancer (in Japanese). Nippon Rinsho 54:1286–1291
23. Makuuchi HE (1996) Ophageal endoscopic mucosal resection (EEMR) tube (in Japanese). Surg Laparosc Endosc 6:160–161
24. Soehendra N, Binmoeller KF, Bohnacker S, Seitz U, Brand B, Thonke F, Gurakuqi G (1997) Endoscopic snare mucosectomy in the esophagus without any additional equipment, a simple technique for resection of flat early cancer. Endoscopy 29:380–383
25. Fleischer DE, Wang GO, Dawsey S, Tio TL, Newsome J, Kidwell J, Prifti S (1996) Tissue band ligation followed by snare resection (band and snare). A new technique for tissue acquisition in the esophagus. Gastrointest Endosc 44:68–72
26. Lee DK, Lee SW, Kwon SO, Jang WI, Shim YH, Cho MY (1996) Endoscopic mucosectomy using an esophageal variceal ligation device for minute gastric cancer. Endoscopy 28:386–389
27. Grund KE (1997) Argon plasma coagulation (APC): Ballyhoo or breakthrough? Endoscopy 29:196–198
28. Shimao H, Hiki Y (1997) Photodynamic therapy for esophageal cancer (jap) Gan To Kagaku Ryoho 6(23):36–40
29. Savary JF, Monnier P, Fontolliet C et al (1997) Photodynamic therapy for early squamous cell carcinomas of the esophagus, bronchi, and mouth with m-tetra (hydroxyphenyl) chlorin. Arch Otolaryngol Head Neck Surg 123:162–168
30. Barr H, Shepherd NA, Dix A, Roberts DJH, Tan Wc, Kranser N (1996) Eradication of high grade dysplasia using 5 ALA and acid suppression: a photodynamic duo. Lancet 348:584–585
31. Overholt BF, Panjehpour M (1996) Photodynamic therapy for Barrett's esophagus: clinical update. Am J Gastroenterol 91:19–23
32. Sampliner RE, Fennerty B, Garewal HS (1996) Reversal of Barrett's esophagus with acid suppression and multipolar electrocoagulation: preliminary results. Gastrointest Endosc 44:523–525
33. Wang KK, Wongkeesong M (1996) A new method of endoscopic treatment for Barrett's esophagus. Gastrointestinal Endosc 44:627–629
34. Ponec RJ, Kimmey MB (1977) Endoscopic therapy of esophageal cancer. Surg Clin N Am 77:1197–1217
35. Lambert R (1998) Endoscopic treatment of esophagogastric tumors. Endoscopy 30:80–93

Quality of Life in Patients with Oesophageal Cancer

J. M. Blazeby, D. Alderson, J. R. Farndon

University Department of Surgery, Bristol Royal Infirmary, Bristol, BS2 8HW, UK

Abstract

There is a growing interest in assessing quality of life in patients with oesophageal cancer because it provides detailed information of the patients' perception of the benefits or harms of treatment. Yet few studies have prospectively measured quality of life using validated appropriate instruments. There are now several questionnaires for patients with cancer, although these are not sufficiently sensitive to small but clinically important changes in quality of life. It is therefore recommended that a disease-specific module is used in conjunction with generic measures. The European Organisation into Research and Treatment of Cancer (EORTC) QLQ-OES24 is currently completing an international validation study. It is used with the EORTC QLQ-C30 core instrument and is designed for patients undergoing potentially curative treatment or palliation of malignant dysphagia.

Studies that have assessed quality of life after oesophagectomy have generally found that survivors do regain their former health. Little is known about the effect of neoadjuvant chemoradiation on patients' quality of life. Following endoscopic palliation of dysphagia, quality of life can be maintained and improvement of swallowing is seen. A validated appropriate assessment of quality of life should be included in future palliative trials and in studies of new treatments which may marginally influence survival but cause significant side effects.

Introduction

Treatment for patients with oesophageal cancer has traditionally been evaluated according to four measurable parameters – mortality, morbidity, survival time and relief of dysphagia. Although improvements are continually being made, most patients still have a poor prognosis, and those who survive may suffer profound physical, nutritional and psychological dysfunction caused by the knowledge of the diagnosis and treatment. Monitoring the quality of life in patients with oesophageal cancer has therefore become increasingly

Recent Results in Cancer Research, Vol. 155

important and can be useful in a number of clinical and research settings. Quality of life data may assist both doctors and patients in decision making. Quality of life questionnaires can be used as screening tools to identify those who might benefit from psycho – social intervention. Quality of life information is vital in the evaluation of new treatments and it is important to health case economics.

What is Quality of Life?

Previously, dysphagia was thought to have the overwhelming influence on quality of life in patients with oesophageal cancer. Most authors have measured swallowing ability assuming it to be representative of overall quality of life [1, 2]. This assumption has been modified by measuring dysphagia grade as well as assessing other aspects of patients' well being [3–6]. The findings have been mixed, but generally indicate that dysphagia is by no means the dominant determinant of quality of life, and a combination of dysphagia, nutrition, performance status and other symptoms as well as social and psychological well-being constitute quality of life for patients with oesophageal cancer. Indeed, the generally accepted medical definition of quality of life, as a multi-dimensional concept should always address at least the core elements of physical, psychological and social well being [7].

Quality of Life Measurement

Standardised methods of quality of life data collection are recommended to minimise missing data. The assessments can be based on observations, interviews or self-report questionnaires. Observations may have to be used if patients suffering from disseminated malignancy are too frail to complete a questionnaire but observer bias and inter-observer variation must be taken into account. Observer-rated quality of life scores do not always agree with those reported by the patients themselves and, thus, observer ratings need to be interpreted with caution [8]. Quality of life data may be collected in a standardised interview by a trained researcher, but patients sometimes have difficulties revealing their true feelings in a face to face situation [9]. It is therefore generally recommended that, wherever possible, questionnaires should be completed by patients themselves. Ideally, a trained interviewer should be available to clarify the question formatting and if necessary help the patient to complete the questionnaire.

Choosing a Questionnaire

It is essential to use a quality of life instrument that is valid, reliable and practical because, without these characteristics, results may be inaccurate, data collection incomplete and information of little clinical use. Reliability and validity testing are performed to ensure the questionnaire is free from measurement error. When choosing an instrument, these details must be checked. Reliability checks include test-retest evaluations, inter-rater reliability testing and internal consistency scores. Questionnaires should be validated by ensuring that the instrument is able to discriminate among patients' subgroups, sensitive to changes in quality of life over time and that the content is appropriate to the specific research question. It is important to ensure that instruments are precise, well laid out and easy to administer and score. Some produce an overall quality of life score, while others yield multiple scores that may influence data analysis. Normal population data manuals are now available for some generic measures of quality of life.

Quality of life instruments may be placed on a continuum reflecting their intended spectrum of application: (1) generic instruments, (2) disease-specific measures, (3) diagnosis-specific measures and (4) ad hoc instruments [10]. *Generic instruments* that cover a broad range of dimension, attempt to measure general health regardless of particular disease and allow for comparison of results across studies of different patient populations. This is an advantage in larger health policy and resource allocation issues. A major disadvantage is that they may be more sensitive to some particular conditions but not others. *Disease-specific measures* are designed for use in homogeneous groups of patients, such as those with cancer. These have similar advantages to generic measures of health, in that they allow comparisons between different groups of patients, but may be insensitive to small but clinically significant changes in quality of life. *Diagnosis- or treatment-specific instruments* are useful because they allow for comparisons to be made between patients with the same malignancy. The obstacle to disease-specific measures, at present, is the lack of reliable and valid instruments. *Ad hoc study measures* have formed the majority of quality of life assessments in the past. Ad hoc measures are simple lists of questions put together without any formal testing. This approach may give quick and easy results, but they often lead to subjective and unreliable data. When choosing a quality of life questionnaire, one solution is to include both a disease-specific and generic measure which will incorporate the positive features of both. This is referred to as a modular approach to quality of life assessment. Using a core instrument (a generic or disease-specific questionnaire) and a diagnosis-specific module reconciles the two requirements of quality of life assessment by providing a sufficient degree of generalisation to allow for cross study comparisons and a level of specificity adequate to address questions of particular relevance to a given group of patients.

Quality of Life Instruments Used in Oesophageal Cancer

In 1977, Stoller et al. published a new proposal for the evaluation of treatment for carcinoma of the oesophagus defining four domains of quality of

Table 1. Quality of life questionnaires used in patients with oesophageal cancer

Questionnaire	Type of instrument	Publications
Karnofsky Performance Scale [14]	Performance scale	McCaughan [12], McCaughan [15], Mahoney [16], Albertsson [17], Flores [18], Flores [19], Reed [13], O'Rourke [20], Herskovic [21], Knyrim [22], Fujita [23]
Eastern Cancer Oncology Group Scale [28]	Performance scale	Mellow [25], Rutgeerts [26], Flores [19], Highley [27]
World Health Organisation Scale [24]	Performance scale	Chavy [29], Sugimachi [30], Flores [18], Baba [31], Baba [32]
Linear Analogue Self Assessment [33]	Cancer specific	Barr [5], Barr [34], Loizou [35], Loizou [6]
Quality of Life Index [36]	Cancer specific	Barr [5], Barr [34], Loizou [35], Loizou [6], Zieren [37]
Rotterdam Symptom Checklist [38]	Cancer specific	van Knippenberg [3], O'Hanlon [57]
European Organisation into Research and Treatment of Cancer [40]	Cancer specific	Ringdal [42], Blazeby [4], Blazeby [8], Blazeby [43], Zieren [37], Bamias [59]
Functional Assessment of Cancer Therapy [39]	Cancer specific	–
Short Form 36 [45]	Generic measure	McLarty [48]
The EORTC Oesophageal Cancer Specific Module [43]	Disease specific	Blazeby [44]
The Visick Classification [49]	Disease specific	Gasparri [50], Barbier [51], Watson [2], Fuchs [52]

life: swallowing ability, work habits, enjoyment of leisure and sleeping habits [11]. Information on dysphagia was considered of paramount importance, with failure to sleep comfortably ranking secondary to dysphagia grade. The questionnaire was completed by an independent observer and has been used by several groups in a variety of clinical situations. No formal reliability or validity data exist [12, 13]. Since this original work, few have examined quality of life in patients with oesophageal cancer and no fully validated disease-specific instrument has been developed. Table 1 shows the English-language publications that have used a variety of questionnaires to measure quality of life in patients with oesophageal cancer.

Performance Measures

Several researchers have evaluated quality of life with simple measures of performance as well as dysphagia grade. This gives more general information about patients' well being, but most performance measures are based on simple observer scores of physical function and, as such, are not recommended for use alone in quality of life assessments.

The Karnofsky Performance Scale

The Karnofsky performance scale is frequently referred to as a proxy measure of quality of life in clinical trials, because it only measures physical function [14]. Despite its inadequacy as a quality of life measure, it is often inappropriately used as such [12, 13, 15–23]. The scale comprises 11 categories ranging from normal performance to death and is particularly weak at accurately measuring quality of life in patients who are immobile due to poor physical health. Such patients may score very low on a physical scale but may be either emotionally or socially well.

The Eastern Cancer Oncology Group (ECOG) Scale

This simple scale looks at performance status and is scored on five points by an observer from grade 0 – able to carry out all normal activity without restriction – to grade 4 – completely disabled [24]. It has not been widely used in patients with oesophageal cancer [19, 25–27].

The World Health Organisation Performance Scale

The World Health Organisation (WHO) five-point scale is physician rated and is very similar to the ECOG scale with the same disadvantages [28]. It has been used infrequently in patients with oesophageal cancer [18, 29–32].

Cancer-Specific Instruments

The linear analogue self assessment scale (LASA) was developed for patients with advanced breast cancer [33]. It has 25 items, ten related to disease symptoms, five to psychological disabilities and five which measure other physical indices. The scale has been validated and tested for reliability, but many patients find it difficult to accustom themselves to representing their feelings on a continuum. It has been used in patients with oesophageal cancer, although it lacks items relating to eating and dysphagia [5, 6, 34, 35].

The Spitzer Quality of Life Index

The Spitzer quality of life index is a simple, short measure of quality of life developed for use in patients with cancer or chronic illnesses, which consists of five items assessing activity, daily life, overall health, support and outlook [36]. It has also been used in patients with oesophageal cancer [5, 6, 34, 35, 37].

The Rotterdam Symptom Checklist

The Rotterdam Symptom Checklist was originally designed to measure the toxicity and impact that treatment for cancer had on psychosocial functioning [38]. It contains 30 items, which can be divided into two primary scales measuring physical and psychosocial disability. An adapted version for patients with oesophageal cancer has been developed in The Netherlands [3].

The Functional Assessment of Cancer Therapy Scale

This 34-item questionnaire (FACT) was developed and tested in an American population and contains four scales addressing physical, social, emotional and functional well being, as well as a scale that considers the doctor/patient relationship [39]. At the end of each set of items assessing a quality of life dimension, a single item asks patients to rate how much that dimension affects quality of life. This scale is reliable and valid and specific modules are available for some disease sites. One is currently being developed for patients with oesophageal cancer.

The European Organisation for Research and Treatment of Cancer Questionnaire

The European Organisation for Research and Treatment of Cancer (EORTC) QLQ-C30 incorporates five functional quality of life scales, a global health scale and three symptom scales. Six single items assess symptoms and problems commonly found in patients with cancer [40]. It was developed with a modular approach in mind so that disease-specific questionnaires could be added to the core instrument [41]. Reliability and validity testing has been extensively performed in several groups of patients including patients with oesophageal cancer [4, 8, 37, 42]. It is available in over 15 languages and an oesophageal cancer-specific module is currently undergoing international validation [43, 44].

Generic Measures of Quality of Life

The Medical Outcomes Study 36-Item Short-Form Health Survey

The Medical Outcomes Study (MOS) SF36 is a self-administered tool that addresses eight conceptual areas of quality of life covering general health, daily activities, work, emotional problems, social activities, mental health, pain and vitality. It has been extensively validated in a variety of patient populations and data are available from the general population [45–47]. It is probably not specific enough to detect small changes in quality of life in patients with oesophageal cancer although it may be useful in long-term survivor studies [48].

Disease-Specific Measures

The EORTC Oesophageal Cancer Module

The EORTC QLQ-OES24 questionnaire module is designed to supplement the EORTC QLQ-C30 core questionnaire [43]. It may be used in patients undergoing oesophagectomy with or without neoadjuvant or adjuvant chemoradiation, patients undergoing primary radiotherapy or chemoradiation and patients being intubated or undergoing endoscopic tumour ablation with laser, diathermy or alcohol injection. It contains six hypothesised scales and five individual items addressing dysphagia, deglutition, eating, upper gastrointestinal symptoms, pain, other specific symptoms and emotional problems relating to oesophageal cancer. No reliability or validity data have been published although it is currently undergoing an international validation study [44].

The Visick Classification

The Visick classification was developed in the 1950s and was designed to assess the outcome of surgery for peptic ulcer disease [49]. It is an observer-rated scale which addresses nutrition, weight loss, dysphagia and regurgitation as well as the ability to enjoy leisure and the ability to work. It has been used in patients with oesophageal cancer to measure quality of life, although it was not designed for this purpose [2, 50–52]. This scale mainly assesses symptoms without considering the psychosocial impact of ill health.

The Effect of Oesophagectomy on Quality of Life

Following oesophagectomy, most patients have some initial difficulty in consuming foods and they may experience heart burn. Patients report that meals take a long time to eat with loss of appetite [2]. Five year survivors claim that appetite eventually returns [30]. Early satiety is another common residual symptom which leads patients to eat small but frequent meals. The effect of a cervical or an intrathoracic anastomosis on functional eating ability has been studied, although how this influences other aspects of quality of life is uncertain. There are no significant relationships between quality of life scores and the type of resection or tumour histology [53]. There is a significant correlation between quality of life scores and relative body weight. Weight loss following oesophagectomy may reflect difficulties in eating, recurrence of disease or psychological problems. Patients who have relatively low body weights or a sudden decrease in weight more than 6 months after oesophagectomy require an intense physical and psychological examination. Others have compared the outcome after oesophagectomy with an intrathoracic anastomosis with that of a retrosternal bypass [54]. The intrathoracic anastomosis causes fewer problems with dysphagia than the retrosternal reconstruction. No significant differences were observed between other parameters of quality of life. The added effect of lymphadenectomy on quality of life and survival has been studied [23]. No differences were observed between three or two field dissection in terms of mortality, morbidity and postoperative quality of life, although patients undergoing three field dissection survived for longer. Most studies show that patients suffer little long-term pain after oesophagectomy [3, 55]. Two-year follow-up data from Bristol using the EORTC QLQ-C30 questionnaire, however, reveal quite different results [56]. All patients reported more pain after surgery. This gradually decreased in those who survived 2 years, although it always remained higher than preoperative levels. This may be explained by the different approaches to pain assessment. Our own study is one of the few in which patients completed the questionnaires themselves. It is not surprising that patients suffer a general decrease in performance and severe fatigue lasting for at least 6 months after surgery [3, 16, 20, 37, 57]. There is a gradual return to normality in those who remain free from recurrence. This profound effect on physical function dramatically influences patients' ability to return to work. Only one-fifth of those working before oesophagectomy are able to continue afterwards, and, after surgery, 67% of patients report a partial or complete incapacity in work or household tasks [30, 37].

The effect of oesophagectomy on psychosocial well being is not fully understood. Roder et al. compared quality of life data following oesophagectomy with a representative random group of the normal population, healthy persons and a group of patients with varying types of malignancy [53]. Loss of ability to socialise caused much anxiety. Another study using the Rotterdam Symptom Checklist reported that psychological function improved following surgery. Zieren et al. asked patients to complete the EORTC QLQ-C30 at the same time as a psychologist completed the Spitzer quality of life index [37]. Only one-third of patients reported emotional disturbances and a decrease in social function. Both studies reported quality of life data from disease-free survivors only. Further quality of life assessments should be performed in patients with problems and recurrent disease because it is in this group that psychosocial support is probably most needed.

The effect of adjuvant chemotherapy or radiotherapy on quality of life is under investigation. In view of the increasing use of both modalities before and after surgery and the associated toxicity with little effect on survival, quality of life data must be a part of the evaluation of new treatments.

The Effect of Radiotherapy on Quality of Life

Flores et al. studied 211 patients undergoing irradiation therapy [18]. Performance improved in those who had started with reasonable pre-treatment scores. In a larger study performance scores, swallowing and weight loss were recorded [19]. Six months after treatment, 56% of patients had improved swallowing performance and less pain. Others have reported conflicting results [20, 58]. Further studies which include assessment of the burden of repeated treatments and hospitalisation are required to fully evaluate the effect of radiotherapy.

The Effect of Endoscopic Palliation of Dysphagia on Quality of Life

Patients undergoing palliation of malignant dysphagia require effective treatment with minimum morbidity and mortality and maximum gain in quality of life. There are many different methods available to relieve the obstructed oesophageal lumen all with similar outcomes in terms of disease-free survival and morbidity, and quality of life is therefore of greatest importance to these patients with limited life expectancy. It can be difficult to assess, however, because patients are often frail, confused or not well enough to be bothered with repeated interviews or questionnaires.

Intubation, the main stay of palliative treatment, continues to be associated with a considerable morbidity and mortality, despite the introduction of expanding metal stents. Immediate respiratory complications, eating adjustments and chest pain may cause long hospital stays and a poor quality of life. Later complications, such as recurrent dysphagia or symptoms of metastatic disease, also impinge on quality of life by requiring repeated hospital admissions. Most studies have only assessed dysphagia as an indicator of quality of life and the few that have incorporated quality of life instruments have only studied small numbers of patients [13, 22, 52, 57]. They generally found that although dysphagia may be improved by intubation, no other aspects of quality of life changed after treatment. In patients receiving treatment with palliative intent, maintenance rather than improvement of quality of life may be the best outcome.

The immediate morbidity associated with endoscopic laser treatment is generally less than following intubation with a plastic prosthesis, although this difference has not been reported to cause a difference in patients' quality of life [5, 25, 26, 52]. Tumour recurrence causing dysphagia, however, is much more common and may require repeated endoscopic follow-up. This is perceived by some (clinicians and patients) as burdensome and disruptive when the inevitable outcome is a short time ahead.

Conclusion

There is a great need to define standard outcomes for patients with oesophageal cancer. An objective assessment of quality of life should be included in future palliative trials and in studies of new treatments which may marginally influence survival but cause significant side effects. Validated self-completion questionnaires should be used wherever possible and the new EORTC QLQ-OES24 questionnaire module to use with the EORTC QLQ-C30 is likely to become the most appropriate instrument after completion of the EORTC international validation study. Data generated from carefully designed trials, employing appropriately chosen quality of life instruments, should improve the management of patients with oesophageal cancer and thus improve their quality of life.

References

1. Earlam R, Cunha-Melo JR (1980) Oesophageal squamous cell carcinoma: 1. A critical review of surgery. Br J Surg 67:381–390
2. Watson A (1982) A study of the quality and duration of survival following resection, endoscopic intubation and surgical intubation in oesophageal carcinoma. Br J Surg 69:585–588
3. van Knippenberg FCE, Out JJ, Tilanus HW, Mud HJ, Hop WCJ, Verhage F (1992) Quality of life in patients with resected oesophageal cancer. Soc Sci Med 35:139–145
4. Blazeby JM, Williams MH, Brookes ST, Alderson D, Farndon JR (1995) Quality of life measurement in patients with oesophageal cancer. Gut 37:505–508
5. Barr H, Krasner N, Raouf A, Walker RJ (1990) Prospective randomised trial of laser therapy only and laser therapy followed by endoscopic intubation for the palliation of malignant dysphagia. Gut 31:252–258
6. Loizou LA, Rampton D, Atkinson M, Robertson C, Bown SG (1992) A prospective assessment of quality of life after endoscopic intubation and laser therapy for malignant dysphagia. Cancer 70:386–391
7. Schipper H, Clinch J, Powell V (1990) Definitions and conceptual issues. In: Spilker B (ed) Quality of life assessments in clinical trials. Raven, New York, pp 11–24
8. Blazeby JM, Williams MH, Alderson D, Farndon JR (1995) Observer variation in assessment of quality of life in patients with oesophageal cancer. Br J Surg 82:1200–1203
9. Bremer BA, McCauley CR (1986) Quality of life measures: hospital interview versus home questionnaire. Health Psychol 5:171–177
10. Aaronson NK, Cull A, Kaasa S, Sprangers MAG (1994) The EORTC modular approach to quality of life assessment in oncology. Int J Ment Health 23:75–96
11. Stoller JL, Samer KJ, Toppin DI, Flores AD (1977) Carcinoma of the oesophagus. A new proposal for the evaluation of treatment. Can J Surg 20:454–459
12. McCaughan JS Jr, Williams TE Jr, Bethel BH (1985) Palliation of oesophageal malignancy with photodynamic therapy. Ann Thorac Surg 40:113–120
13. Reed CE, Marsh WH, Carlson LS, Seymore CH, Kratz JM (1991) Prospective, randomised trial of palliative treatment for unresectable cancer of the oesophagus. Ann Thorac Surg 51:552–556
14. Karnofsky DA, Burchenal JH (1949) The clinical evaluation of chemotherapeutic agents in cancer. In: Macleod CM (ed) Experimental cancer therapy. Columbia University Press, New York, pp 191–205
15. McCaughan JS, Nims TA, Guy JT, Hicks WJ, Williams TE, Laufman LR (1989) Photodynamic therapy for oesophageal tumours. Arch Surg 124:74–80
16. Mahoney JL, Condon RE (1987) Adenocarcinoma of the oesophagus. Ann Surg 205:557–562
17. Albertsson M, Ewers SB, Widmark H, Hambraeus G, Lillo-Gil R, Ranstam J (1989) Evaluation of the palliative effect of radiotherapy for oesophageal carcinoma. Acta Oncol 28:267–270
18. Flores AD (1989) Cancer of the oesophagus and cardia: overview of radiotherapy. Can J Surg 32:404–409
19. Flores AD, Nelems B, Evans K, Hay JH, Stoller J, Jackson SM (1989) Impact of new radiotherapy modalities on the surgical management of cancer of the oesophagus and cardia. Int J Radiat Oncol Biol Phys 17:937–944
20. O'Rourke IC, McNeil RJ, Walker PJ, Bull CA (1992) Objective evaluation of the quality of palliation in patients with oesophageal cancer comparing surgery, radiotherapy and intubation. Aust NZ J Surg 62:922–930

21. Herskovic A, Martz K, Al-Sarraf M, Leichman LP, Brindle J, Vaitkevicius V et al (1992) Combined chemotherapy and radiotherapy compared with radiotherapy alone in patients with cancer of the oesophagus. N Engl J Med 326:1593–1598
22. Knyrim K, Wagner HJ, Bethge N, Keymling M, Vakil N (1993) A controlled trial of an expansile metal stent for palliation of oesophageal obstruction due to inoperable cancer. N Engl J Med 329:1302–1307
23. Fujita H, Kakegawa T, Yamana H, Shima I, Toh Y, Tomita Y et al (1995) Mortality and morbidity rates, postoperative course, quality of life, and prognosis after extended radical lymphadenectomy for oesophageal cancer. Ann Surg 222:654–662
24. Zubrod CG, Schneiderman M, Frei E, Brindley C, Gold GL, Shnider B et al (1960) Appraisal of methods for the study of chemotherapy of cancer in man: comparative therapeutic trial of nitrogen mustard and triethylene thiophosphoramide. J Chron Dis 11:7–33
25. Mellow MH, Pinkas H (1985) Endoscopic laser therapy for malignancies affecting the oesophagus and gastroesophageal junction. Arch Intern Med 145:1443–1446
26. Rutgeerts P, Vantrappen G, Broeckaert L, Muls M, Geboes K, Coremans G et al (1988) Palliative Nd:YAG laser therapy for cancer of the oesophagus and gastroesophageal junction: impact on the quality of remaining life. Gastrointest Endosc 34:87–89
27. Highley MS, Parnis FX, Trotter GA, Houston SJ, Penson RT, Harper PG et al (1994) Combination chemotherapy with epirubicin, cisplatin and 5-fluorouracil for the palliation of advanced gastric and oesophageal adenocarcinoma. Br J Surg 81:1763–1765
28. World Health Organisation (1979) World Health Organisation handbook for reporting results of cancer treatment. WHO, Geneva
29. Chavy AL, Rougier M, Pieddeloup SA, Kac J, Laplanche AC, Elias DM et al (1986) Oesophageal prosthesis for neoplastic stenosis. A prognostic study of 77 cases. Cancer 57:1426–1431
30. Sugimachi K, Maekawa S, Koga Y, Ueo H, Inokuchi K (1986) The quality of life is sustained after operation for carcinoma of the oesophagus. Surg Gynecol Obstet 162:544–547
31. Baba M, Aikou T, Natsugoe S, Kusano C, Shimada M, Kimura S et al (1997) Appraisal of ten-year survival following oesophagectomy for carcinoma of the oeosphagus with emphasis on quality of life. World J Surg 21:282–286
32. Baba M, Aikou T, Natsugoe S, Kusano C, Shimada M, Nakano S et al (1998) Quality of life following oesophagectomy with three field lymphadenectomy for carcinoma, focusing on its relationship to vocal cord palsy. Dis Oesop 11:28–34
33. Priestman TJ, Baum M (1976) Evaluation of quality of life in patients receiving treatment for advanced breast cancer. Lancet i:899–900
34. Barr H, Krasner N (1991) Prospective quality-of-life analysis after palliative photoablation for the treatment of malignant dysphagia. Cancer 68:1660–1664
35. Loizou LA, Grigg D, Atkinson M, Robertson C, Bown SG (1991) A prospective comparison of laser therapy and intubation in endoscopic palliation of malignant dysphagia. Gastroenterology 100:1303–1310
36. Spitzer WO, Dobson AJ, Hall J, Chesterman E, Levi J, Shepherd R et al (1981) Measuring the quality of life of cancer patients. A concise QL-index for use by physicians. J Chron Dis 34:585–597
37. Zieren HU, Jacobi CA, Zieren J, Muller JM (1996) Quality of life following resection of oesophageal carcinoma. Br J Surg 83:1772–1775
38. de Haes JCJM, van Knippenberg FCE, Neijt JP (1990) Measuring psychological and physical distress in cancer patients: structure and application of the Rotterdam Symptom Checklist. Br J Cancer 62:1034–1038
39. Cella DF, Tulsky DS, Gray G, Sarafian B, Linn E, Bonomi A et al (1993) The Functional Assessment of Cancer Therapy Scale: development and validation of the general measure. J Clin Oncol 11:570–579
40. Aaronson NK, Ahmedzai S, Bergman B, Bullinger M, Cull A, Duez NJ et al (1993) The European Organization for Research and Treatment of Cancer QLQ-C30: a quality of

life instrument for use in international clinical trials in oncology. J Natl Cancer Inst 85:365–376
41 Sprangers MAG, Cull A, Bjordal K, Groenvold M, Aaronson NK (1993) The European Organisation for Research and Treatment of Cancer approach to quality of life assessment: guidelines for developing questionnaire modules. Qual Life Res 2:287–295
42. Ringdal GI, Ringdal K (1993) Testing the EORTC quality of life questionnaire on cancer patients with heterogeneous diagnoses. Qual Life Res 2:129–140
43. Blazeby JM, Alderson D, Winstone K, Steyn R, Hammerlid E, Arraras J et al (1996) Development of a EORTC questionnaire module to be used in quality of life assessment for patients with oesophageal cancer. Eur J Cancer 32:1912–1917
44. Blazeby JM, Alderson D, Farndon JR, Conroy T, Arraras J, Hammerlid E et al (1997) An international field study to test the EORTC QLQ-C30 and oesophageal cancer module (EORTC QLQ-OES24) among patients with oesophageal cancer. Protocol no 15961/40973
45. Ware JE, Snow KK, Kosinski M, Gandek B (1993) SF-36 Health survey manual and interpretation guide. New England Medical Centre, Boston
46. Jenkinson C, Coulter A, Wright L Short form 36(SF36) health survey questionnaire: normative data for adults of working age. Br Med J 306:1437–1444
47. Garratt AM, Ruta DA, Abdalla MI, Buckingham JK, Russell IT (1993) The SF36 health survey questionnaire: an outcome measure suitable for routine use within the NHS? Br Med J 306:1440–1444
48. McLarty AJ, Deschamps C, Trastek VF, Allen MS, Pairolero PC, Harmsen WS (1997) Oesophageal resection for cancer of the oesophagus: long-term function and quality of life. Ann Thorac Surg 63:1568–1572
49. Visick AH (1948) A study of the failures after gastrectomy. Ann R Coll Surg Engl 3:266–284
50. Gasparri G, Casalegno PA, Camandona M, Dei Poli M, Salizzoni M, Ferrarotti G et al (1987) Endoscopic insertion of 248 prostheses in inoperable carcinoma of the oesophagus and cardia: short-term and long-term results. Gastrointest Endosc 33:354–356
51. Barbier PA, Luder PJ, Schupfer G, Becker CD, Wagner HE (1988) Quality of life and patterns of recurrence following transhiatal oesophagectomy for cancer: results of a prospective follow-up in 50 patients. World J Surg 12:270–276
52. Fuchs KH, Freys SM, Schaube H, Eckstein AK, Selch A, Hamelmann H (1991) Randomised comparison of endoscopic palliation of malignant oesophageal stenoses. Surg Endos 5:63–67
53. Roder JD, Herschbach P, Sellschopp A, Siewert JR (1991) Quality-of-life assessment following oesophagectomy. Theor Surg 6:206–210
54. Kuwano H, Ikebe M, Baba K, Kitamura K, Toh Y, Matsuda H et al (1993) Operative procedures of reconstruction after resection of oesophageal cancer and the post operative quality of life. World J Surg 17:773–776
55. Bluett MK, Sawyers JL, Healy D (1987) Oesophageal carcinoma. Improved quality of survival with resection. Am Surg 53:126–132
56. Blazeby JM (1998) Quality of life in patients with oesophageal cancer. MD thesis, Bristol University
57. O'Hanlon D, Harkin M, Daya K, Sergeant T, Hayes N, Griffin SM (1995) Quality of life assessment in patients undergoing treatment for oesophageal carcinoma. Br J Surg 82:1682–1685
58. Sawant D, Moghissi K (1994) Management of unresectable oesophageal cancer: a review of 537 patients. Eur J Cardiothorac Surg 8:113–117
59. Bamias A, Hill ME, Cunningham D, Norman AR, Ahmed FY, Webb A et al (1996) Epirubicin, cisplatin, and protracted venous infusion of 5-fluorouracil for oesophagogastric adenocarcinoma. Cancer 77:1978–1985

Subject Index

Recent Results in Cancer Research

Volumes published since Vol. 146

Volume 146
Rectal Cancer (1998)
ISBN 3-540-63544-0
P. M. Schlag (Ed.)

Volume 147
Isolated Liver Perfusion in Hepatic Tumors (1998)
ISBN 3-540-63336-7
K. J. Oldhafer, H. Lang, R. Pichlmayr (Eds.)

Volume 148
Assessing the Economic Value of Anti-Cancer Therapies (1998)
ISBN 3-540-64030-4
N. Neymark

Volume 149
Bisphosphonates in Clinical Oncology (1998)
ISBN 3-540-63689-7
B. Thürlimann (Ed.)

Volume 150
Fast Neutron and High-LET Particles in Cancer Therapy (1998)
ISBN 3-540-57632-0
R. Engenhart, A. Wambersie (Eds.)

Volume 151
Cancer Chemoprevention (1998)
ISBN 3-540-64710-4
H. J. Senn, A. Costa, C. Jordan (Eds.)

Volume 152
Adjuvant Therapy of Primary Breast Cancer VI (1998)
ISBN 3-540-64085-1
H. J. Senn, R. Gelber, A. Goldhirsch, B. Thürlimann (Eds.)

Volume 153
Peptides in Oncology (2000)
ISBN 3-540-64429-6
K. Höffken, R. Kath (Eds.)

Volume 154
Genes and Environment in Cancer (1998)
ISBN 3-540-64430-X
M. Schwab, H. Rabes, K. Munk, P. H. Hofschneider (Eds.)

MIX
Papier aus verantwortungsvollen Quellen
Paper from responsible sources
FSC® C105338

If you have any concerns about our products,
you can contact us on
ProductSafety@springernature.com

In case Publisher is established outside the EU,
the EU authorized representative is:
Springer Nature Customer Service Center GmbH
Europaplatz 3, 69115 Heidelberg, Germany

Printed by Libri Plureos GmbH
in Hamburg, Germany